MY NAME IS SHARON

Printed and Electronic Versions
ISBN: 978-1-7354093-6-8
(Dominick Domasky/Motivation Champs)

The book was printed
in the United States of America.

To order additional copies or bulk order contact the publisher, Motivation Champs Publishing. www.motivationchamps.com

When this ambiguous grief
Grabs ahold of thee,
Know our love
Is what keeps me free.

These arms that used to hold you tight
and slay bed monsters late in the night
Are now grateful during this unscheduled role
In which you hold me, in your memories so
close.

The lights may have dimmed
But I am still here.
I hear the words you whisper in my ear.

Souls eternally bonded,
This world can't tear us apart.
Forever connected between our mirrored hearts.

E.W. Rightings

INTRODUCTION

From as far back as I can remember, my mom was there for me. Every time my mother volunteered at the school, corrected my obnoxious behavior, drove me to the orthodontist, or wrote a kind note to one of my teachers, she was doing it for me. Not as a helicopter parent, or to run my life, but out of love. One hundred percent pure love.

With two children of my own, I have learned that parenting is a complex and challenging journey. For my mom, the journey was no different. I surprised Mom by being born two months early, so I tested her from the start. She always reminded me that I was born with a full head of hair. I think as a beautician, that brought her pride. As a child, I struggled with my speech and the basics of school, but Mom wouldn't dare let me fall behind. She helped with my lessons, science projects, and volunteered religiously at the school. As a teen, I pushed boundaries and many times challenged my mom's authority. Her belief in me never wavered. She stood strong and kept me from going off track. Mom and my sister had their clashes, too, but it was all out of love. Mom was doing her best.

I'm so grateful for my mom's unconditional love. Looking back on our lives together, the love and kindness she shared were magical.

Many of us never get a chance to say goodbye to our

parents. The end comes suddenly, and we're left with the burden of what we wished we had said. My mom is alive, but I worry I've already missed my opportunity. My mother has dementia, and she's been robbed of her memory and past memories. It's not fair, but illness and loss never are.

If I could go back to before things changed, I would. I'd thank her for the sacrifices she made. I'd say, "I love you." I'd make sure she knew I meant it. I'd apologize for any grief or worry I caused and promise to be better. I'd hug her so tight and never let her go. Life doesn't work that way, though; there are no redo's. Even with our greatest efforts, we only get to play the hand we are dealt.

Mom was dealt a cruel hand. She no longer recognizes the grandchildren she once adored. Children she gave her heart to are now strangers. The gold band she wears on her left ring finger "belongs" to a man who visits often but always leaves brokenhearted.

Even with heavy hearts, unconditional love is what my mom shall receive. In a lifetime of effort, never could I equal the amount of love my mom so naturally graced me with.

My mother is my hero, and these are her memories.

MY NAME IS SHARON

CHAPTER 1

THE GUARDIAN

—

SUMMER 1986

Sitting in my parents' black, mid-eighties Oldsmobile Cutlass, I stared out a slightly cracked window and watched my mom cross the narrow blacktop street and disappear into the local corner market. The building had a suspect appearance. Its exterior was a putrid yellow, dirty siding, and its front was aged, with fog-covered commercial glass doors. The market was a rundown house converted into a corner store. Above the door hung a sign that read Paul's Store, and like this local spot, it had seen better days.

None of that mattered, though, because it was Mom's go-to for warm loaves of the fresh Italian bread that my sister, Dad, and I craved. Bread this fresh, you immediately had to reach into the paper bag and start tearing off chunks to enjoy. Mom would get mad about the crumbs dropping in her car, but she let it slide just to see us smile.

As I sat there awaiting my flaky treasure and playing with my rubber wrestling action figures, a group of teens took notice of me and my looks (or lack thereof). The typical insults of the day were shared, but it was nothing I hadn't heard before. The car doors were locked, and I was as safe as I needed to be. WrestleMania was already in full swing, so I continued using the dashboard to re-enact an epic duel between Hulk Hogan and King Kong Bundy.

Before long, Mom was on her way back with two white bags, each containing a loaf of that coveted Italian bread. Mom never appreciated nonsense, so she quickly shooed the teens from around her car. Upon entering, she rolled down her window, and I followed, using my twig-like arms to wind mine down. At that very moment, seizing his opportunity, a brown-haired teen decided to spit through my open window. The side of my face was his target, and he accomplished a big, slimy direct hit.

Whether or not he caught a death stare from my mom, I do not know, but I do know he ran for his BMX and pedaled like hell.

Mom slammed her car in reverse, then into drive, and created a gravel shower peeling out of that parking lot. The kid had broken rule number one, messing with my mom's children—and he was going to pay. The kid turned left, Mom turned right. It was like Mom had a homing device on the kid and knew his every move. She tore up one narrow street and down another, never slowing to check where the boy might be. It was as if she already knew.

In an instant, we were face-to-face. The teen looked at us like he had seen a ghost and let his bike fall to the street. He took off running toward his friends in the adjacent park. My mom stopped the car in the middle of the street (and left me in the car) to pursue the fleeing teen. You've heard the term "Dad Strength." Well, this was "Mother Speed." Within seconds, she was upon the boy's friends. They stood frozen, offering no help. They parted, and Mom caught her target cowering near a brown fence. I could see her talking and him nodding. She didn't raise a fist, or her voice, but whatever she said, it hit home.

The teen turned away from my mother, and as his friends looked on, he walked to our car. He stepped over his bike and signaled for me to lower my window. I timidly did as he requested. The teen apologized and extended his hand. I leaned out the window and reached out my arm, and peace was made. He picked up his bike and walked toward the park.

Mom never mentioned the incident again, not to me, Dad, or my sister. To my mom, protecting her family was as natural as breathing; she didn't need anyone's validation.

CHAPTER 2

LOOKING FOR CLUES

—

PRESENT DAY

I'm no longer a little boy. Decades have passed and roles are reversed; it is my turn to defend my mother. I find myself at my parents' house searching through Mom's packed dresser drawers and file cabinets. All so full they bow upon opening. Mom's Alzheimer's has grown severe, and today she's in a home. I'm looking for account numbers, passwords, and any other information that could potentially help with her care. It is like trying to find a needle in a haystack, except that I don't know what the needle looks like. The haystack is a house full of receipts, memories, and more I'm sure to uncover.

Mom kept a lot of stuff over the years, but as her illness progressed, she hung on tighter to memories. By trying so hard to hold on to so much, I wonder if it allowed a lot of important things to fall through the cracks. Searching for answers has become akin to putting a puzzle together. Every paper I find provides a new clue, and each picture unlocks a memory. This process takes months, but I'll do whatever I have to do to make sure Mom gets the care she needs. I also find myself with the responsibility of sharing her story. I owe it to her.

Together, we'll embark on this journey, and we'll do it one photo, document, and memory at a time.

Here's one, my sister and I are lying on the floor with our grandparents. I'm about three years old with pudgy features and a shag haircut. My sister is six, with straight bangs and a formal blue and red dress. We're hanging out by an ashtray on the floor and all have cigarettes in our mouths. Everyone is smiling—those were different times.

More pictures of my grandparents—Mom's parents. Pictures of their home in Las Cruces, and pictures of us all enjoying time together. Pictures of Mom as a little girl playing with her younger brother and the neighborhood kids. Mom and her brother were less than a year apart, so their mom often dressed them as twins in their early years. Mom let me know *many* times she wasn't a fan of that.

Born in Roswell, the well-known site of the alleged 1947 UFO crash, Mom and her family moved to Las Cruces, New Mexico, shortly after her father got a job at White Sands Missile Base. Mom grew up just fifty miles from Mexico in a town that still feels like what America's suburbs were meant to be. It's quiet, and people say hello to their neighbors.

Another box. What's this I see? A school progress report. "Dominick is struggling to hear and repeat his vowel sounds." I had to take remedial reading and speech classes all through grade school, and progress reports like these are just some of the things Mom saved.

"Thank you for the apples," one teacher wrote. "Thank you for your efforts with the Parent-Teachers Association," another signed. Mom was always at the school, volunteering and helping. Why couldn't I appreciate it back then?

I have children, and I'm so proud of them, but Mom cared so much about my development that she kept all my report cards and progress reports.

"Dom is still having some difficulty making vowel sound association. However, he has improved since last grading period." —Miss Knopf, Report Period 2, Kindergarten.

"Dominick needs reinforcement to apply skills. He sometimes becomes frustrated. He can usually do it." —Miss Miliotis, Grade 1.

"Dom's present grade is a 63 percent. This now puts him in serious jeopardy with respect for passing the course for the year." —R. Albright, 5/1/1996, senior year.

Before cellphone photos and social media posts, Mom was already magnificently documenting our lives.

There were photos of our Thanksgiving costumes. Mom dressed my sister and me up like Pilgrims, and man, were we mad. Mom sewed costumes so we could participate in our elementary school's Thanksgiving Day party. I had buckles on my shoes, long socks, and a tall, black hat. My sister had a long dress, pigtails, and her outfit was completed by funny socks and shoes to match. Our classmates made fun of us—and it hurt—but no one had made them costumes.

When I threw my retainer away in the cafeteria garbage, Mom drove to the school to help me sort through the trash. When I did it again, Mom was there. She even knew what color napkins she had packed in my lunch, so while I stalled (and often gagged), Mom easily navigated the saucy plastic plates and chocolate milk-covered trash.

Mom was always by my side, no matter how messy things got.

Things are messy here too. We learned Mom had been opening accounts and moving money for years. I learned of this when a bank called me for overpayment regarding an account I never knew I was on.

CHAPTER 3

NUMBER ONE
EMPLOYEE

——

PRESENT DAY — REMEMBERING

My search continues, and I scan an intimidatingly full bookshelf in Mom's bedroom, formerly my sister's room when we were kids living at home. Some thin papers stuck out from the top of a book on Greece: "Icon's Restaurant and Grille" it read. Mom had stowed away two gift certificates she'd purchased from me when I owned a restaurant: purchased, but never redeemed. Mom always found a way to help.

"Mom, drop thirteen pieces of fish and one basket of fries," I called. This is restaurant shoptalk. I was asking Mom to put breaded fish and french fries into a fryer.

Unpredictable business and multiple employees calling off for one shift: that was a normal day when I owned the restaurant. The good news was Mom often passed through to drop off homemade desserts. These weren't for me to eat; they were for me to sell.

I opened my own restaurant at twenty-three. Although

I was young and underfinanced, I made a go of it for a few years. Mom did things like wash the aprons and pitch in where she could. When my business started to struggle and things crashed around me, she often offered a lifeline. Many days she worked in the hot kitchen manning the fryers. Other days she took charge of the dishwashing station. She cleared grimy plates and worked with purpose, inspecting each dish to make sure it met her high standards. Other days, when I got a rush of business at an off-peak time, she greeted guests and made them feel appreciated.

Everyone's favorite thing was her desserts. When money got tight and I could no longer bring in enough ingredients to make those quality confections, Mom stepped in. She made fresh desserts on her own dime, in her own kitchen, and she brought them to the restaurant for me to sell.

Key Lime, Caramel, and Oreo Cheesecakes; fresh pies and elaborate chocolate cakes—you name it, Mom made it. Mom's desserts were made from scratch, and she learned to bake out of love. Her son's business was struggling, and she wanted to help. She didn't stick twenties in my pocket or bail me out; she did more than that. She let me be me and had my back. She didn't seek the limelight or keep score; she was just there for me. She went above and beyond, just as she had back when I was her little boy, whether being spit on by a teenager or struggling to hear my vowel sounds—Mom showed the same vigilance protecting me, even as an adult.

She was so proud and supportive when I decided to chase my dreams and open a restaurant. She helped me paint the walls and frame over a hundred pictures. A few months before we opened for business, I was able to invite her as a guest to our first food tasting. In an attempt to win our business, we were invited by Sysco Food Service, a national food purveyor, to their test kitchen, and they prepared my entire menu. Together we enjoyed their cooking and a special day. When we opened, she helped in any way she could, from dropping fish into the fryer, seating guests, or making runs across town for products. She was there when I closed, too, offering support and encouragement for my future—which she still believed was bright.

There were tough times, and my restaurant failed, but I was never alone. My mom was there to experience it all. From start to finish she lifted everyone's spirits when she walked through the front door, always—including me.

CHAPTER 4

SPOIL THEM ROTTEN

—

2006 – 2013

Mom loved my kids so much. Behind her back, my wife and I called her Nanny Claus, because every time she visited our children she came bearing gifts. I worried she'd spoil them. Would they end up terrible people if they were always getting gifts?

One day a week, she watched my son during the day. They were always doing something special. First it was my son she spoiled, but after a few years, our daughter was born and joined the party too. Without considering the dirty diapers (they were a handful), Mom never complained. She read them books, took them to unique places to play, the library, matinees, and always made sure they had soft blankets for naps.

The books that made them smile, she read over and over. *Everyone Poops* was always a favorite. My children were obsessed with flipping through the pages, and it had them in stitches every time. Mom didn't mind their raucous amusement. When the books became worn, she repurposed them with a mastery of clear tape.

—

After about nine months of watching both my son and daughter together, Mom started saying my son was drinking a lot of water—more than usual. She repeated her concerns while we were recognizing the same thing at home. Long after bedtime, he would leave his room and descend our creaky steps. As young parents finally getting ten minutes to ourselves, we'd encourage him to return to bed, but to no avail. He'd hit the kitchen to chug a thirty-two-ounce Gatorade, and we'd tell him to slow down. The drink would be empty, and he'd complain he was still thirty. Soon my three-year-old son was at Pittsburgh's Children's Hospital, hooked up to machines and tubes. His blood sugar was over eight hundred, and the doctors confirmed he was diabetic.

My wife and I stayed at my son's bedside for three days, and our daughter stayed with my mom. Mom was glad to be her granddaughter's caregiver, and my wife and I continued pretending to be strong. From that point forward, Mom seemed to be a little more protective of Madilyn.

When Mom and Dad visited the hospital, she carried a pen and a pad. Regardless of who entered the room, candy striper or endocrinologist, Mom's pen was in action. She was always a diligent notetaker, but those days it was more. A yellow Post-it note hung on the dishwasher, *clean dishes*. By the telephone, a white card taped to the wall and written in cursive, *Dom's cell*, *Alissa's home*, *Richard's cell*, and *shop phone* (which was my dad's nursery of forty-five years). In the basement, in thick black marker, *Keep door shut!* Outside of the basement, on the door to the inside, *Do not open, cat's inside.*

Diabetes added confusion to her days with the kids, but she did her best. She helped my son prick his finger for blood and tracked all of his daily glucose readings. Mom tried so hard to understand the basics of diabetes, but it never really set in.

Learning new things was becoming harder. When cell phones went android, she tried to make the transition. Her cellular provider convinced her to buy a phone with a touchscreen, but Mom just swiped and swiped. She was never able to make a call and returned the phone. She was comfortable with her tiny red flip phone. A few years later Dad tried buying her a bigger, better one, but the results were the same.

I saw signs, but made my share of excuses, trying to justify what was happening. When it involved the safety of my children, my eyes were opened. Measuring and administering insulin shots was just too much to ask. My wife would sneak out of work on her lunch break or I'd change my schedule to be close. Mom had always protected her children with vigilance, and I needed to do the same.

CHAPTER 5

MY LITTLE HELLIONS

—

SUMMER OF 2014

Mom continued to watch my children, but as they grew more rambunctious, Mom was at her limit. Spilled juice cups and backtalk got her excited, but horseplay really set her off. If nonsense happened during a trip in the car, everything escalated. Having been taught by the best on how to protect a child, I started limiting how much Mom and the children would be in the car together. I'd try to eliminate her need to drive or ask my dad if he could help. Always willing, Dad did what he could.

Regardless of our best-laid plans, life happens in its own way. Mom was watching my children, and my son had to get to his baseball game. The location was at Polish Town, a baseball field on a hill near my house that had seen better days. Mom had taken me to many games at that field and cheered me on there when I played youth baseball. The parking lot was a hilly grass lot full of tree stumps and bent signs. Mom ended up being their driver and called for details. I tried to ease concerns by explaining it was the old field I played on just a few streets from my house. I figured there would be no issues, and we ended the call.

Seconds later I received another call; it was Mom. We went through the same conversation, as if we hadn't just talked. Calling right back was not atypical for her; however, most of the time it was to confirm additional details or tell me another story. But this was different. She was confused and disoriented. We had moved across town four or more years before that day, yet she kept asking about my old address.

"Near the bakery?" she asked. "By the firehall?" she questioned.

"No Mom, in Youngwood. I don't live in town anymore," I responded. "The field over by where we adopted the dogs." Near the ball field was a home that I'd hoped she'd remember. As a boy, she and I went there together, and she'd allowed me to adopt not one, but two dogs. Predator and Madonna were their names—Weimaraner and Lab mixes—and she and I loved those dogs. Neither the dogs nor the home rang a bell.

With the help of my children and another call or two, she made it to the field. My phone rang. Another call from Mom, "We're here. Cameron just ran up to the field."

After the game, Mom couldn't find her way back to

my house. She called a few times saying she didn't know where to turn, each time getting further from both of our houses. I blamed my kids—they were probably acting up—so I dismissed her confusion and rerouted her back in our direction. I didn't want to face the truth. Mom always came through.

A few minutes later she pulled into my driveway, and our children were buckled tight. As usual, they were safe. Mom was superwoman, and I was her defender. On that day, I excused what happened. I told myself it was my children's behavior and the fact that I had moved a few years prior. I made up all kinds of excuses to avoid the truth. We all did.

CHAPTER 6

CHANGING ROLES

—

2015–2017

During a phone call or an in-person visit, Mom would tell a story about her cats or somewhere new my sister had vacationed, and moments later we'd hear the same story again.

At first, I responded with something like, "Mom, we just talked about that." After a few times, you lose patience. My mom was too young to be losing her memory. She had to be tired or not paying attention. There had to be a reason, a fixable cause for this. Mom's too organized too. Nothing is wrong. Scared to hurt our loved ones, we tell ourselves *it's just me noticing*, but then you ask others close to you, and they're noticing things too.

I asked my sister about Mom's memory, and she noticed a change as well, saying, "We always talk about the cats," or "Mom told me the same story about the kids three times."

But some noticed nothing.

—

"Your mom looks like she's doing great," they'd say.

Others wanted to feel better about their bond with Mom and chose to ignore the signs.

"We talked for a long time. She always knows me" is another response I heard.

They were wrong. More and more people confirmed what I was witnessing. We talked to Dad, and he was seeing signs too. Household activities and responsibilities Mom once tended to were now being ignored. Dad was there morning and night, and he experienced all my mother's trials and tribulations firsthand. After forty-five years, he and my mother switched roles, and now Dad was the primary caregiver. Dad became domesticated— his cooking improved, he took over laundry duties, and became Mom's driver.

These oversights and misses started seeping into his business too. For forty years while Dad was out on job sites, Mom masterfully handled billing and payables. She documented everything, filed it her way, and controlled every detail from distributing gas cards to quarterly taxes. As Mom's Alzheimer's progressed, Dad had to work double-time to uncover where things went off track. The deeper Dad looked, the more twisted the web became.

I thought we could work together and get Mom to go to the doctor. We all agreed there was probably some kind of medicine that would help her memory, like a magic pill. We all want a magic pill at some point. Everyone forgets things; maybe Mom was just working too much. She helped an elderly woman a few days a week and watched my children a day or so, and that's a lot for anyone.

When I reached out to my uncle, her brother, and asked him if he noticed anything, he replied, "She's probably just tired," and "Sure, she repeats herself a little bit."

My concern continued to rise, so I contemplated approaching Mom.

First you try being subtle, slipping it into a conversation. "Some of my friends' parents take medicine to help their memory; did you ever think of doing something like that? I know I would if the doctor would prescribe it."

She didn't bite.

When I had more courage I tried being more direct. "Mom, maybe you should see a doctor. I think you're starting to forget some things."

She'd snap: "I'm not forgetting anything," and follow with an aggressive, "Maybe you don't need my help."

Any mention of memory loss was met with rage. Her mother, who we affectionately called "Shebby," had battled Alzheimer's as well. Maybe that weighed on her more than she let on. My sister would send letters to Mom from Texas and make calls recommending the same. We were both met with resistance. Mom would show a level of aggression we seldom saw growing up. This level of anger rarely surfaced, but my sister and I recognized it.

This anger was something my sister and I experienced when we committed the worst of teen offenses. My cooking teacher called the house because I was acting up and being disrespectful in class—I was actually hiding from a kid named Tom behind the teacher's knife drawer—a forbidden spot, but my safest circle of protection. I may have been able to argue my way out of that, but when the teacher gave me detention and I responded with "I'll kill you," I was in *big* trouble. Mom's head nearly exploded when I got off the school bus and walked into the house.

My sister feared these explosions as well. Once she tried to fool Mom by adding a few percentage points here and there on her report card. Mom caught her a few months later, and I still smile knowing it was her and not me who received Mom's wrath. Only in her children's worst moments was Mom as angry at us as she was at the suggestion of memory loss.

That teenager who spit on her son, he saw it too.

With the help of Dad and my sister, we tried for

years to get Mom to chat with her doctor, but we failed over and over. We tried the subtle approach, then being straightforward, and we attempted trickery. Above all, our loved ones deserve dignity, so there were lines we couldn't cross. You can't force someone to do something they're unwilling to do. Mom put up more of a fight every time we tried.

I'm filled with regret: *Why wasn't I a better son? If only I could have been more persuasive, or maybe I should have picked her up and carried her over my shoulder. Then we could have put her in the car, driven her to the doctor, walked her into the office, and had her checked out. Then the doctor would have agreed with us and immediately diagnosed her condition. After that, he would have placed her on game-changing medicine, which she would take religiously, and she would be healed.*

Things are not that simple. This was no fairytale, and Mom was on a different journey. She was scared. Now I pray her moments of realization are few.

CHAPTER 7

FADING AWAY

—

SUMMER 2018

Mom loved her cats so much. My parents lived in a farmhouse on the outskirts of town, and for some reason, those dumping unwanted cats must have found its peaceful appearance appealing: white split rail, a classic American wooden barn, and rose bushes, a welcoming location for any animal in need of a second chance. Mom, with her heart of gold, took in stray cats. She showed them love. She made sure they were fed and taken to the veterinarian regularly. She didn't allow them inside, so she had cat boxes built and filled them with blankets to help the cats stay warm. She even covered their opening from the elements by stapling some fabric or carpet over the doors.

For as long as I can remember, we always had cats: Samantha, Animal, Dr. Doom, Lucky, Calli, Oreo, Lightning, and more than I know after I moved out. They'd walk back and forth on the back deck purring and looking for food. Sometimes they'd bring mice from the barn to show Mom they were worthy of her love. She approved too. What she didn't approve of was another cat or animal being mean to the cats she cared for. If Mom caught wind that one of her cats was getting picked on, she became defensive.

"Get the hell out of here!" she'd yell.

I tried to share how vigilantly Mom protected me, and her cats were no different. If a raccoon or possums got aggressive, she'd stop whatever she was doing and leap into action, chasing the wild animal off with a broom.

Once I had children, Mom got a little softer with her rules and started bringing a few cats inside. She broke her thirty-year rule to make my little ones smile. She let my daughter name a cat "Peanut," and when my daughter visited, they played together in the basement. When it was cold, my mom allowed another inside. The cycle continued. Then Mom began to worry that none were safe outside if one was in a fight. She brought more inside, and before long, there were more notes too. *Don't open the door.* Or *Shut the door tight; there are cats inside.*

Mom watched my dogs when we went on vacation: Rocky, Rosie, and Juliette. Rocky was a pug I bought for my wife before we had children. Mom loved Rocky and showered him with toys and treats. If we went away, she'd take Rocky on walks and sit in the backyard with him and have what she referred to as a picnic.

After Rocky passed, Mom watched Rosie when we

went away. Rosie was a mix of Beagle and Bulldog, and Mom loved her too. Rosie was only around a short time and passed from eating a poisonous mushroom. Her sudden death left loneliness at our house, and soon we found another shelter pet that needed a forever home. Our new dog's name was Juliette, and she was a mix of Pitbull and Terrier. Juliette, who had a gimp leg, was a sweet dog that just wanted to be loved.

Mom thought Juliette was a good-looking dog but never really remembered her name. One of the things we noticed with my mom's memory loss was new things were forgotten first. New phones, new people, or a new pet's name just didn't stick with her memory. New experiences were lost immediately.

To save a few dollars on kenneling, I asked Mom to watch Juliette while we took a trip. She had enjoyed it in the past, so I convinced myself it was okay. By this point, I knew I needed to confirm it with my dad, and he was fine with it too. My mom wrote it on her calendar a few weeks in advance, and I called every few days to remind her.

She said, "Just let me know the day before, and I'll move the cats."

That was how she handled it; she'd move the cats from one basement room to another.

The night before our trip and the day of Juliette's visit, I called again: "Mom, can you move the cats?"

Mom said, "When are you coming?"

I replied, "Tomorrow." And on the next day's call I said, "Two hours."

When I arrived, I walked Juliette around the back of the house and into a mudroom in the basement. Things seemed kosher, so I took Juliette off her leash and double backed outside to chat with my dad. As my dad and I shot the bull, I started to hear barking and ruckus coming from inside. It escalated quickly, and the barking grew louder and more frequent. I went to investigate. Upon opening the door, I witnessed half of Juliette's body in the cathouse. The box was rocking back and forth, and there were all kinds of wild noises filling the room. I pulled Juliette by her hips. Both cat and dog rolled out onto the linoleum floor. The dust spraying everywhere reminded me of an old-school cartoon battle where both characters morphed into one big, rolling tumbleweed.

Neither the cat nor Juliette were backing down, and my standing was doing little to help. I took a leap of faith and entered the tumbleweed. I may not have rolled across the floor with them, but afterward, I sure felt like I'd gotten tossed around. I was able to get Juliette outside, and I went back for the cat.

I made a quick stop to ask Mom about the cat, but this wasn't a good day. She hadn't moved any of the cats and wasn't sure how many were inside. My plan for a quick drop off was foiled.

I rustled all the remaining cats into the next room and went back outside to retrieve Juliette. I filled her bowl with food and headed into the laundry room to fill her water bowl as well.

"Shit," I said, when I heard more barking. Juliette was trying to squeeze herself behind Mom's large deepfreeze. I had a bad feeling. When I slid myself on the deepfreeze and looked on the other side, another cat. Another crazy day, but these were becoming the new normal.

When we got back from vacation, none of the zip-locked bags of dog food were gone, and Juliette's bowl was full of cat food. This was our new normal with Mom, and the last time I asked her to watch Juliette.

CHAPTER 8

OUR LAST
THANKSGIVING

—

NOVEMBER 2018

It wasn't long before we couldn't let Mom drive anymore, and by that point, she really didn't mind. This is a woman who had cruised the Caribbean islands, visited Spain, Greece, Hawaii, traveled the country, Canada, and South America. Her memory was slipping, but she was still with us 60 percent of the time. During those times, she loved telling us about her high school majorette team and marching in the Rose Bowl Parade. Her school took buses across the Southwest for the big event.

Another of her favorite subjects was going to school and being friends with Alden Tombaugh. His dad was Clyde Tombaugh, the man who discovered Pluto. Mom was invited to their house for dinner a few times too. Drop "My friend's dad discovered Pluto," into any conversation, and my mom instantly had the floor. When I was in elementary school, Mom suggested I do a report on Pluto. Without me knowing, Mom made a call and pulled some strings. Before my report was due, Alden

Tombaugh sent me a nice letter and some of his dad's artifacts. I got an A on the project for my exemplary planetary knowledge.

Back on planet earth, Mom's driver's license had expired, and she didn't fight too hard to reapply. In Pennsylvania, the laws stated she would have to retest, and I think she wanted to avoid that. She always felt free behind the steering wheel, proudly telling me about when she and her friend Phyllis used to sneak their parents' cars out at night and drive fifty miles from Las Cruces and over the border into Mexico for a fun night. I soaked up those stories, but there were fewer and fewer. More and more she wasn't with us. I could see her start to drift. Either she was quiet or would randomly speak up about things that did not apply.

"Ha, ha, ha . . ." smiles and chuckles, her laugh. It would boom loudly, out of nowhere.

When she was with us, she repeated herself constantly, and by this time we were all witnesses to her decline.

My dad thought it would be nice to plan a grand Thanksgiving dinner, an epic feast at their house where Mom didn't have to lift a finger. It would be a holiday to remember.

Their intentions were pure, but by this point, Mom craved routine. Dad and Sis invited the whole family, my in-laws and all. They planned every detail, from the seating to the disposable silverware. We had more food than you could imagine. The whole thing was catered, and there was something for everyone. Even if you were on a mission to overindulge, it would have been hard to locate all the options.

Mom contributed where she could, warming buns and corn in the microwave, but it was my dad and sister who didn't miss a single detail. We pulled tables into the family room and lined both sides with guests. We laughed, smiled, watched football and, of course, ate pie.

It was a beautiful day together, and everyone was filled with joy and turkey. The meal was a success. The whole family pitched in, and in unison, we cleared the table while complaining about our glutinous ways. My niece and nephew played in the barn with my children, so any rowdiness remained out of sight. The sun was setting, and as always, it beautifully framed my parents' backyard. Their yard was full of green grass, large maples, oaks, and evergreen trees dancing throughout. In the distance lay the woods, and above them, a cornfield I ran through as a boy. Dusk was coming, and darkness too.

Mom started acting different, worried, distrustful. It was like nothing I had seen. She wanted us to get her car, and she wanted to go home. Mom was disoriented. To me, it felt as if she didn't recognize her home.

She headed toward the front door and wanted to leave. She asked for her keys and looked out toward the spot where her car typically sat. Ever since she quit driving, her gray car was parked in the driveway in front of the house, but on that day we moved it so our guests could park closer. When Mom looked out her door, things were different.

She wanted us to call Richard, but Richard (my dad) was sitting in his recliner. None of us were familiar to her, and soon her fog turned to panic. Mom wanted things back the way they were, and so did all of us. I hugged my mom as tight as I've ever held her and asked everyone to put things back as they were. No one argued or offered suggestions. My family came together. We moved furniture, packed food, and put her car and house back in place.

We fixed what we could and parted ways. We had now seen a new side of Alzheimer's and dementia, and it was progressing fast.

CHAPTER 9

MAGICAL MOMENTS

———

CHRISTMAS 2018

Holidays came and went, and gone was the innocence of the past. Not long ago, my main holiday concern was if my mom was spoiling my children too much. Now, I anguished over whether or not she would remember their names when they approached her for hugs. It's hard to explain memory loss to a child. Only experience makes coping easier; however, no child should have to face the ugliness of a loved one's memory slipping away.

When I was a boy, I had so many toys. I often think back and wonder how my mom wrapped and positioned so many presents under the tree for Christmas morning. Many of us have tiptoed in silence and wrapped presents on holiday nights. How did our parents do it with such ease? For my wife and me, our hearts were beating out of our chests—our timing was never quite right. No matter how quiet we tried to be, floors creaked and doors squeaked, or it was time for a nightly bathroom break. Every year, I feared waking my children and crushing their spirits.

———

My mom, though, she was magical. No matter how late I stayed up or where my sister and I snooped, we never found a present. Christmas morning, stockings hung full, and perfectly wrapped gifts lined our living room. My parents worked hard, but they were not rich; however, on Christmas Day you'd believe otherwise. We spent hours opening presents, and it always felt like there was one more tucked away.

Mom also made our favorite dinners. Mom made me, my sister, and my dad each our favorite dinner. Three separate meals. However, that wasn't the case anymore. Now we celebrated at Mom and Dad's on Christmas Eve. One year, the presents weren't wrapped, and she went upstairs for hours. By the time she came back, my children were sleeping. Another year, when we showed up Mom was working late caring for an elderly woman. There was no dinner as suggested, so we ordered Chinese food.

In 2019, there was nothing, not even a tree. Dad worked long hours at his snow removal business, and he tried his best. He bought us each a card, but this year he had to sign my mother's name.

CHAPTER 10

TWISTED MEMORIES

—

PRESENT DAY — REMEMBERING 2019

A Stephen Curry bobblehead still rests on the mantle at my parents' house. Mom loved the way he smiled, played with flair, and paraded across the court with his mouthpiece hanging out. I used to love Michael Jordan the same way. I had the shoes, drank the Gatorade, watched his games, and tried to mimic his every move.

On the day I got cut from the seventh grade basketball team, I remember walking down our gravel driveway after school. Mom was waiting for me as she looked out the front door in excitement. When I could see her, I put my finger to my throat and ran it across my neck. I wish I hadn't been so callous. Getting cut from the basketball team hurt, but I know it hurt my mother more. Years later, when I made other teams or accomplished something special, she would always remind me of that day. Mom believed you never wanted to get too high or be too low.

We had a lot of talks on that porch. Talks about hoops, college, friends moving away, and uplifting conversations when I felt lost. Mom was tough, but she was the kindest when we needed it most. Always a listening ear.

When I was cut from the team, my mom bought me a pass at the YMCA and drove me to town anytime I wanted to play. I fell in love with its dusty courts and became a student of the game. I made the team the next year and never got cut again. I never had to ask, but my YMCA pass was always renewed. Because of her support, I was able to make team after team and even played in college. Mom was always in the stands.

Before most of her memory was lost, Dad took her to Philadelphia to watch the Warriors and Stephen Curry play. When I saw them a few days after they came back from Philly, Mom had a wonderful story about meeting Stephen Curry. She said, "He was the nicest man." I was absolutely floored! How could neither of them call me and tell me this? I was freaking out.

I asked, "Did you get his autograph?"

Her reply, "Yeah, we had lunch, and he wrote me a letter."

At this point, the basketball fan in me was about to lose my mind, so I looked at my dad and asked him about the incident.

Dad looked at me and softly said, "None of that happened."

Having spent nearly a decade watching my mom battle this disease, I know now that it happened in her mind. To her it was *real*. There was no need for me to correct her or try to prove it didn't happen. That would be cruel.

My dear friend, Eric, once shared with me some sage wisdom in regard to caring for a loved one with advanced memory loss. He had been by his grandmother's side during her battle with Alzheimer's and comforted me with the following words:

"When you were a baby, even though you couldn't talk or understand what your mother was saying, she still held you, talked to you, and cared for you. Why? Because you needed it. Now, even though what she's saying may not make sense, and she may not understand you, it is your duty to be there for her as she was for you."

Eric's advice has comforted me so much during this journey, and I feel a responsibility to share his words with others whom they may help. I'm sorry his grandmother struggled, but I am grateful he shared this message with me.

I'll never question or judge the words my mother now says. I'll offer eye contact and reply with love. *Mom, please know this: I'm listening*.

CHAPTER 11

GUILT IS A HEAVY WEIGHT

—

2019 PREPARED US FOR 2020

Maybe I could have done more; maybe I should have tried harder. It took years for us to get Mom to visit a neurologist, and I regret the time lost. Maybe we could have slowed the spread of the disease, but if we brought up memory loss, Mom was ready for a fight. If we persisted, she held a grudge. To my dad, I can only offer gratitude and love for all those late nights and early morning battles he fought alone.

Attempts to speak with my mom's doctor were always difficult. HIPPA guidelines don't allow the sharing of medical information, and Mom was not sharing either. Sometimes Mom would add my sister and me as contacts on her medical forms, which gave us snapshots into her records; then on her next visit, she would remove us. When we called with concerns, we were constantly told by medical personnel, "You're not listed as a contact anymore." The more Alzheimer's stole from her, the more secretive she became. She held on to some memories longer than others, so adding that to her defiance when questioned by a doctor, and she was hard to diagnose.

A doctor would ask, "Is this your son? What's his name?"

And she'd reply, "I know his name; why don't you tell me what the hell his name is?"

Time kept slipping away, and so did Mom. Finally, out of desperation, I walked into my mother's doctor's office at noon and pleaded my case to the medical staff. I had prepared a handwritten note expressing my concerns, and I asked them to hand it to the doctor. The receptionist asked me to be seated, and I waited alone. A short time later, the staff member walked out and guided me to an exam room. The doctor had agreed to see me.

She didn't offer files but expressed so much compassion and concern for Mom. She had cared for my mother for years and was quite fond of her. She alluded that Mom had missed more than half of her appointments over the last few years. She cared about my mom's well-being, and it was apparent. She shared that she had suggested my mother see a specialist regarding her memory, but Mom had canceled the appointments. The doctor was also adamant about my mother adding us to her privacy forms, but we know how that was going. She also wanted to make sure my dad brought her and was in the room for visits.

The doctor had confirmed what we were seeing. Upon hearing this, my sister, my dad, and I worked our way into every medical conversation and appointment.

My mom never liked the first neurologist. I met him while selling pharmaceuticals, and he was strongly recommended, but Mom said he tried to touch her inappropriately. In cases of accusation, my dad would *always* counter her with the truth, because he had been in the exam room as well. Each time a test was suggested, or Dad would try to get Mom to an appointment, she had a unique defense system: either she wasn't ready, refused to get up, or would just throw a fit. Because of this, she was able to miss more and more appointments until she made it emphatically clear she would not see that doctor again.

So we searched for another doctor, hoping that maybe they would be the one that could help my mom get better. My sister made the calls and spent hours researching options. Soon we had another appointment with the next neurologist. For the first visit, I met Mom and Dad at the office. Mom was cordial but surprised to see me in the waiting room. When the medical assistant called her name, we all stood, but she said she was going in by herself. Dad spoke sternly and said he was going in too.

They entered without me, but I wasn't raised to give up so easily. I went to the receptionist and told them I wanted to be in the room too. They understood, but needed to run it by my mom and dad. Mom agreed. On my way to the exam room, I was able to meet the doctor and speak freely with him. I spoke bluntly and shared intimate details of my mother's condition. Dad didn't have to speak in code to get his concerns across to the doctor, and neither of us had to worry about offending my mother.

Once in the room, the doctor asked all the usual questions, and Mom did pretty well. This is what made the disease so tough. She was able to answer the basics like her name, city she lived in—and if she didn't know the answer, she would fire back with her own question.

Slyly, Mom would say "I don't know; what day do you think it is? Why don't you tell me how many kids I have."

Putting people on the defense was my mom's best defense. My dad and I looked at each other like "What now?" Even at her best, she entered a fog every few minutes. If the doctor witnessed it, it would be clear.

"Mom, tell him about the time you met Stephen Curry," I suggested.

My mom immediately told an elaborate story about Stephen Curry. She then topped that one with her time working for Oprah and cutting her hair.

She added, "Oprah was so nice and paid really well."

The doctor was engaged and impressed with my mother's brushes with fame. He actually leaned in, eagerly wanting to know more.

He turned to me and asked what I had once asked: "Is this true?"

Sadly, I shook my head no. I had heard it all before.

CHAPTER 12

AN UNAVOIDABLE PROGRESSION

———

JANUARY 2020

"Dominick, you need to get over here." Those were the ominous words of my father, and they chilled my bones.

When our parents reach a certain age, unexpected calls from them at untraditional times tend to raise the heart rate. My mom hadn't called me for years, and by midevenings Dad was typically in a deep state of relaxation on his favorite chair.

Mom slept more and more these days. It was as if her mind was going into hibernation. Some days I'd pass through in the morning and others in the afternoon or evening. Most days she was sleeping and had become harder and harder to awaken. A good day was a few minutes of coherency usually over a meal. If you asked Mom if she was hungry, it was always no; however, if you unwrapped a chicken sandwich or veggie sub and put it on her plate, she ate it all.

———

Mom was so thin and weak, a shell of her former self. A one-time proud beautician, she could no longer do her hair. Her hair was often messed and matted, and things we all do daily were no longer routine. For most of my life, I had rarely seen my mom wear the same outfit twice, but now the jackets, hoodies, and sweaters felt all too familiar.

After forty years of benefitting from Mom's extraordinary care and homemaking, my father was now thrust into the role of primary homemaker and Mom's primary caregiver. While owning a landscape company and working six days a week, he made the time to take her to appointments, wash clothes, and learn to cook. Dad's first try at pasta, he prepared a whopping five pounds of spaghetti for him and Mom. I saw it firsthand. Still on the counter, with the sauce mixed in, and in a pot so large it looked like something more suited for deep-frying a turkey.

Dad was burning the candle at both ends, not to mention what he must have been going through emotionally. He and his business were collateral damage of a disease that took no prisoners. We did what we could to assist and offer support, whether that meant checking up on Mom during the day or bringing dinner when we could. I think what Dad enjoyed most were the calls and visits from the grandkids. If it was a phone call, we'd talk business, or I'd ask for parenting advice while sharing stories of the wild things my children were up to. During visits, more business and talks about entrepreneurship was always a favorite topic of ours. The kids, though, they wanted Pappy and demanded Old Maid or chess. For a short time, a sense of normalcy.

Our efforts were nothing but a small plug in a leaking dam. Mom was a shell of herself, and Dad's job was becoming more complex. Slips in the shower, falls down steps, kitchen mishaps, wandering, all growing concerns. Mom and Dad needed more help. We met with multiple agencies, and they each promised results. Each time we saw a light, red tape brought us back to reality.

Dad hired various healthcare workers. Some didn't show and others fell asleep on the job or were no match for my mother's advancing dementia. Mom wasn't going to let them tell her what to do or when to do it. Housekeepers tried, too, but for most, the situation was out of their league. Mom's disease made her hide clothes, food, mail, and so much more. Her suspicion and distrust toward us grew greater every day. And her looks of spite are forever burned into my mind.

Sundown brought Sundowners, and when Mom was disoriented, everything was compounded. It wasn't her fault, Dad's, or anyone else's. It just sucks, and there was no right answer. Even with a team approach, dementia continued to win.

Mom would have hated living this way. I know it because her mom battled severe memory loss as well. My mom's lifelong friend, Phyllis, recently shared with me that she and my mother had spoken about dementia.

My mom said to her, "I'm never going to get that."

Phyllis offered encouragement, but she worried for my mother too; she saw signs. The two had been friends since they were little girls, and she knew Mom better than anyone.

We all worried, but there was nothing that could have stopped that ominous call from Dad.

"Dominick, you need to get over here."

Dad was distraught. I tried to get clarity: "What's going on? I need to know what I'm walking into."

"I can't get her up. Something isn't right," Dad replied.

Full of worry, I grabbed my things as calmly as I could—trying not to alarm my children—and I rushed from the house. They had seen too much, and that was my fault. My wife knew things were bad and offered strength.

I had traveled that nine miles hundreds of times, but this time I didn't know what to expect. All normalcy was gone. I was traveling into the abyss. I've studied positivity for over twenty years, however, I couldn't think of a good outcome. Maybe I could put everything I've learned together for one moment and make everything right. Mom would recognize me and I'd save the day.

If only we could write every story. But I wasn't the author and neither was Mom. Dementia was deciding her fate, and this time it was cruel. Mom was sprawled out, laying back, barely on the couch. How she was supporting her weight, I do not know. Her body was contorted with her legs extended out, heels barely touching the floor. I spoke louder and louder, and eventually she opened her eyes. These weren't the results I expected.

I envisioned lifting her up as she had done for me so many times. I'd carry her to a warm bubble bath, fix her a sandwich, and make everything right. Not this time though; I didn't have my mother's touch.

When I tried to reposition her, she swatted my hand away. When I tried to cradle and lift her, she screamed in pain. We tried comforting her by washing her softly with a warm washrag and soap, but she wasn't coming to. We were failing her.

Mom needed help that neither of us could provide, so we called 911. We knew it was the right thing to do, but our hearts broke, knowing the care she required meant she was never coming back home.

CHAPTER 13

CHANGE IS INEVITABLE

—

JANUARY 2020 CONTINUES

Emergency services took the details and quickly sent out an ambulance. I met them in the front yard, and they came around the side of the house with a stretcher. Dad and I moved furniture and stuff to make room, and they started to care for Mom. Her heart rate was high, and they had numerous concerns. They asked us questions, and we did our best to reply.

The paramedics were professional and delicate, treating Mom with dignity and respect. Even with all their training, they could not stop Mom from letting out a call of agony while lifting her onto the gurney. Off to the hospital they went, and Mom was gone.

No one was allowed to ride in the ambulance, so Dad grabbed Mom's purse. We turned the house upside down, hunting for everything we thought she might need: slippers, socks, shirts, pants, undergarments, a toothbrush, insurance cards and, most importantly, her purse. She always loved her purses, and we knew if she had one to hang on to, she'd definitely be more comfortable with that familiar piece of her life.

We scurried to our cars, and I followed Dad. He followed the ambulance. Dad parked in front of the hospital and rushed to the door. I chose the lot below and walked the fifty yards through the bitter January cold. Upon entering, night security had Dad emptying his pockets. They swiped a wand across him, and it beeped while crossing his chest. He had left home in such a hurry, he'd forgotten to remove his pocket knife. After some chaos, security opened some doors and led us down long hallways filled with patients. With each turn, the anxiety grew. Finally, in a room with three walls and a wide open curtain, there was Mom wrapped in an oversized wool blanket. She was still sleeping, even though she was connected to beeping monitors and machines by a complex arrangement of wires and tubes.

I think back to when I was a boy, and Mom never got sick. This woman, lugging dog food bags and all, had always been tough. When I was in ninth grade, she started working at the local thrift store and never missed a day. I think after ten years of perfect attendance she received a plaque. Mom got up early and stayed up late. She'd vacuum at midnight then find more to do. A wonderful blend of kindness and toughness. She rebounded basketball shots for me. She also proudly reminded me of the days when she carried a fifty-pound bag of dog food over each of her shoulders—from the trunk of her car to the bottom of the barn. The dog food story was one of her favorites and quite an impressive feat. She could make enchiladas and cut hair. Writing thank-you notes and making people feel special was a gift she always shared.

Even in the hospital corridors, I was stopped by people who had been impacted by my mother. As an adult, this had become a regular occurrence. People often introduced themselves then told me what a wonderful person my mother had been to them. They'd tell me about her handwritten thank-you notes, the gifts she gave to make them feel special, what a friend she had been, and always how much she loved my sister and me.

One of my aunts said, "We always loved Sharon. You know how sometimes you don't get along with your sisters-in-law or at times you want them to leave? That was never the case with your mom."

The stories of Mom always warmed my soul—for a moment—and then I'd be reminded of her struggle. Mom was hurting, and I couldn't do anything about it. In this case, Mom's heart was racing, and she wasn't responding well. A few doctors seemed to think it was her body shutting down. After a few days, there were still no answers. Despite the dementia, Mom had been in pretty good shape. She was fit, and if she saw me stretching, she often volunteered to touch her toes.

"Did she fall?" a cardiologist asked.

"She always says she fell," I answered.

We never knew how the fall happened. Nor did we know what happened in between my visits, caregiver stops, or when Dad was away. Dad couldn't know what Mom was doing while he was sleeping. This disease didn't rest; it attacked 24-7. Mom had always stayed up late, but now she was awake and wandering. One night Dad heard voices and found my mother in a full conversation. She was talking to the woman in the mirror. If she fell when Dad was at work or when the help wasn't around, who could be sure it really happened?

I explained to the doctor that Mom was tough—and she proved it again. After days in agony, X-rays found that Mom's hip was broken near the joint. It was as if the femur had been cut away with a barbaric tool. That explains her contorted body on the couch, her shriek when I tried to move her, and her racing heart since the injury.

The hospital was where Mom needed to be, and it would be a long road ahead.

CHAPTER 14

EXTENDED STAY

———

MID–JANUARY 2020

Mom's spirits lifted when we walked in the hospital room, which filled our hearts with joy. Before Alzheimer's, she found *something* to compliment in everyone who visited. And to her credit, I believe she was eternally sincere. If I'm labeled as optimistic, then it was Mom who created my sunny disposition.

"Did you get taller? Have you been lifting weights?" Mom would ask.

If I arrived for an afternoon visit in a suit, she'd say "You always look nice, professional, handsome," or compliment my tie.

If I was wearing a bright pair of sneakers, Mom was in her glory. Even as she lost her memory, bright shoes always caught her eye.

Mom loved radiant colors. She had a state-of-the-art kitchen (when it was built in the late '80s) with vibrant green countertops and white cabinets with green fea-

———

tures. The appliances were black, and the room had short green carpet similar to a putting green. The decorations were bold and from all cultures. Mom loved Mexican and African culture. Dolls in bright dresses, artwork, and trinkets depicted stereotypes of the South. Mom had no malice in her heart; she only saw beauty in culture.

When I was a young boy, I idolized Michael Jackson. I collected magazines and articles with his picture on them. I tried to emulate "The King of Pop." I wore pants with lots of zippers and a coat to match. Mom signed me up for breakdancing, and I even had a sparkling silver glove. I listened to his songs over and over, and the "Thriller" video scared me every time. Michael turning into a zombie still makes my heart skip a beat.

When I was sad because I couldn't be more like Mike, Mom was there. I remember fretting, "His skin is so much darker than mine; maybe I can never be like him." Mom didn't want us to be sad, so she found an article that showed his makeup, and said, "See, he's just like you." I didn't know black and white until years later. With Mom, there was only love; and that's how it should be.

Such a special woman, and lying broken in a hospital bed doesn't do her justice. Doctors, nurses, and hospital staff judge my mother for how she reacts to their care and her pain. She lashes out at them when their care hurts, and I see them whisper to each other. I wish they knew the woman I knew, full of compliments and a giver of gifts. They don't.

I watch a staff without empathy manhandle my mom. She resists, moans, and causes a fuss. They ask us to leave, and timidly my wife and I head to the hallway.

After a minute, Mom's frightened and calls my name, "Dominick!" I'm shocked and crushed. I wasn't there for her. Mom had only said my name twice in the last five years, and both times were during her hospital stay. There were times I felt like she recognized me, but not that I was Dominick, her only son. Instead, I was some type of acquaintance. This day was different.

I immediately ran to her in those moments, and the emotions were hard to bear. Both times, medical staff had asked her to do things that obviously made her scared. When she called out, what made her think of me? My friend, author, and holistic healer, Joel Holc, talks a lot about love and fear. He says, "The two can't exist in the same place." If this is true, then hopefully the moment Mom called my name in fear, she was immediately filled with reciprocated love.

CHAPTER 15

WHO ARE WE
TO DECIDE

LATE JANUARY 2020

Days ticked away, and January was coming to an end. Mom had transferred from the hospital to a facility that provided occupational therapy. She had a roommate named Doris who listened to every conversation and kept her television on full blast. Doris still had her memory, but no family nearby. Mom was struggling to adapt but did well with recovery. In no time she was trying to walk out of the building. Purse in hand.

Her stay in occupational therapy was only temporary, and it was time to make a decision on a permanent home. We chose a lovely place where Mom would get the care she needed, and we would be nearby. We did our best to ease the transition. My sister visited from Dallas and arranged Mom's room just as she liked it. She packed my mom's favorite blankets, knickknacks, and family pictures.

After a few weeks in the hospital, Mom was moved

---

to a live-in rehabilitation center. This meant our family was given a few extra weeks to figure out where Mom would go next. Home was no longer an option. Even if we could get Mom some live-in help, my parents' farmhouse had far too many steps, stairs, and trip hazards. A decision needed to be made, and we were running out of time. Trying to make decisions like this while emotionally drained is not something I wish on anyone. Unfortunately, this is all too common.

Mom was safe in rehabilitation. Their team made sure she ate, bathed, changed her clothes, and took her medicine. With a village, they were able to care for Mom. It was evidently clear Mom needed this type of care full time. Mom, who had looked out for all of us, needed more help than we could provide.

Choosing twenty-four-hour care for a loved one is a complex issue. Some have prepared contingency plans, and others hope they're never faced with these decisions. My mom's dementia progressed far too fast to get her input on the issue. When we started noticing her memory loss, it was not a topic she was willing to discuss.

When family, doctors, nurses, dietitians, banks, and bill collectors ask us to make decisions on behalf of our loved ones, we do our best; but what qualifies any of us to make these decisions?

"Mom likes fish and doesn't eat peas." "She would want

her own room, and she'd be fine with sharing a bath-room." "Mom would want a vaccine," and "No, she does not want extraordinary measures to be taken." All these I've said.

There's always the question of whether or not someone knows when they are losing their memory. In looking through her files and documents, I get clues that Mom had an idea of the direction her mind was going. Inside of random books, there were clipped and highlighted magazine articles about memory loss hidden away. Be-hind a pile of clothes is a book about Alzheimer's. Then there were Mom's notes to herself and Dad, notes on the calendars, notes on drawers, shelves, the dishwasher, and strategically placed as a reminder to lock the doors.

When my sister got the room ready, it looked just like home. Mom had all of her favorite things—except for her cats—and was quick to tell you what was hers. She had pictures, dolls, and purses. Dad was there every day, morning and night, helping to ease the transition. The move was probably just as hard on him. He was exhaust-ed but relentless in caring for Mom.

Some days Mom slept through our visits, and some days she needed additional care. Terrible things happen when your brain is shutting down, and everyone did their best to help. We couldn't fight the process, and we didn't delude ourselves anymore. Instead, we accepted it and tried to make it as easy as we could on Mom. While Mom was safe, eating and becoming comfortable with her new home, the painful thing was that often she didn't engage with us. She was quiet and a shell of herself. It was like watching her die from the inside out.

CHAPTER 16

A NEW VIRUS

EARLY FEBRUARY 2020

As February came to pass and March neared, there was talk of a virus. A *new virus*. It was in a faraway land; however, the media seemed to be covering it more and more. Nothing to fear; love was in the air. It was Valentine's Day, and by coincidence, Dad, Liz and I all arrived to visit Mom at the same time.

We brought Mom a pink and blue slushy. She was usually captivated by the colors. Dad came with Russell Stover chocolates, always her favorite. Mom's new home was full of life, and we were led into an activities room full of colorful books, games, and nostalgic pictures. When Mom and I went for walks during visits, this room offered a new experience every time.

On this day, we crowded around a table and made heart-shaped and love-inspired crafts together. A group of volunteers sang songs while Mom sipped on her slushy. Another resident encouraged Mom to stir her drink because he didn't like the way the blues and pinks were separating. She swirled it with a straw. My highlight was when one of the volunteers offered my dad a cookie and enthusiastically told him how nice his Valentine's card was. She didn't realize Dad wasn't a resident. Mom was having a good day, and we had smiles all around. Moments like these made it all feel like this was working. We could do this.

But another day I stopped by to visit, and an Elvis impersonator was on the way. I could see Mom was interested in the commotion, so I led her to a seat in the back. I thought the view was fine for casual observance, but Mom was only interested in the open seats up front.

"Who's sitting in those seats?" she asked.

I thought up some reasons to stay in the back. Maybe we could talk. I tried some of my usual conversation starters, but Mom's attention never wavered from the seats. This wasn't about me. Before Elvis arrived, I walked Mom, arms intertwined, to the front. She got her seat. Mom was content, and I faded out the door.

In March, a few cases of the virus popped up in the USA. I think two people had it in a nursing home out west, so Mom's nursing home proactively posted a notice saying "No One Under Eighteen Allowed." Another sign taped to the door said "Do Not Enter" and had specifics about temperature and travel. I called the number and no one answered. I walked through the entrance doors, punched in the code at the next double door and began entering as I always had. I was in a reception area with an empty desk and a thick daily visitor log. Only one more alarmed door between me and my mom.

"Get out, get out!" a lady with a mask stormed out and shouted.

Her fury was not unwarranted, but I was still caught off guard. I froze. This was pre-COVID, premask, pre-shutdown, precarnage, and I just wanted to see my mom. My delay only made the woman angrier, and she backed me through both sets of doors. I was confused, worried, and stuck outside the building.

"Wait here!" she exclaimed, pointing to a bench by the door.

I sat for what seemed like forever and called again. No answer. *Maybe something was wrong.* My agitation grew. I waited and waited, and finally the caregiver opened the door. She was softer but firm. After explaining the governor's orders, I was appreciative and thankful for her vigilance; she was committed to keeping Mom safe. She explained the new requirements and filled me in on what she knew. She held up what looked like a white plastic gun, and for the first time during COVID, my head was scanned for a temperature. I passed the temperature check and was welcomed in.

I visited with Mom, and I wish I could tell you about

the meaningful conversation we had, but nothing stood out. Everything was surface level, weather, or what movies were on. She couldn't remember anything and couldn't connect to any deeper or meaningful conversation. If only I had known this would be my last visit with my mom before the world shut down, I would have tried something new, something different, anything to connect with her.

I said goodbye and buzzed myself out. When I got to my car, I called my dad to share the news and redirect him. Dad had volunteered to take my son to boxing, and they were planning to stop by afterward. Now they couldn't; no one under eighteen was allowed in.

The next day, there were more confirmed cases. The Seattle nursing home that had one of the first confirmed cases was overrun by COVID-19. Within hours, I received a call from a nurse at my mom's home letting me know there would be no more visitors; they were on lockdown.

CHAPTER 17

FEAR OF THE UNKNOWN

MID-MARCH 2020

On March 13th, 2020, President Trump declares a national emergency. In the days that followed, our country was in chaos, and we were all attached to our television screens. Schools began sending students home, and businesses that were deemed nonessential were forced to close. We were in a global pandemic.

What does that even mean, a global pandemic? We soon found out. Grocery stores were wiped out and people panicked. Not only could we not visit Mom, we couldn't get toilet paper either. The world was in fear and people began hoarding everything from soup to sanitizer. Shelves were bare, and the essentials were being rationed. Some stores reduced hours, and others held special shopping hours for those with the highest risk. We even had a coin shortage. The death toll continued to rise.

I wanted to see my mom—we all did—but the world was on lockdown. Weeks passed, then months, but

COVID-19 didn't go away. The silver lining was that Mom was safe. Her nursing home's stringent policies kept the virus out. Some people believed social distancing and wearing masks helped prevent the virus from spreading, and others felt their civil liberties were being violated.

The country was divided, and social media provided a forum for daily battles. While the country was being torn apart the virus took no prisoners. Unlike Mom's Alzheimer's, a disease that primarily attacked those over fifty-five, COVID attacked us all: healthy, sick, rich, and poor. The president said the virus would be gone by Easter. We hoped with spring and summer, and the return to warmer weather, that we could visit Mom outside. For every step forward, there were two steps backward.

Twenty-twenty was also an explosive year for race relations. Many alarming and unfortunate instances of violence took place between police officers and men and women of color. Often people were asked to choose a side between black lives and blue lives. This type of polarization would have broken my mother's heart, and I was grateful she was spared this pain. She grew up with a military father in New Mexico in the 1950s and '60s and had a diverse upbringing. Her friends were people of color, white, and Hispanic, and her favorite singer was Richie Valens, a crush she would carry for life.

Mom never, *ever* acted privileged—and she had ample opportunity. Her dad worked for the government, her mother served as a legislator, and her parents had a membership to the country club. Her father liked to golf. None of that mattered to Mom. She saw the good in people and not their skin color. She raised my sister and me to be open-minded and compassionate. She often told us stories about traveling as a teen with her brother to Kansas and across the South. Each Summer, the two went by bus to visit their grandparents. After passing through many southern bus stations, Mom often spoke of the separate water fountains for the white people and for those of color. This is when my mom learned of segregation and the impacts of Jim Crow laws. She despised what she saw.

So much has changed in the world, but we still have a long way to go. People deserve better. My mom does too; she would have hated 2020.

CHAPTER 18

NO END IN SIGHT

END OF SPRING 2020

"Rise and shine, Mr. D - O - M! Rise and shine." So many days my mother woke me up with this cheery call. I must confess, it didn't exactly feel cheery in that moment.

I had a bedroom covered with laminated Michael Jordan posters and unique memorabilia, and Mom supported my collection. She was always thinking of others. Seldom did more than a few days pass without Mom surprising me with a new magazine featuring MJ or a collectible like a Wheaties box with his picture on it. Mom thought of others 24-7, and now it had been months since we had seen her. I needed her to know we cared about her too.

Quarantine was a word we all came to know. The elderly were most at risk, and it was decided that the ones in homes were mandatorily quarantined. Hospitals, jails, and many other institutions were the same: no visitors allowed in or out. All employees were temperature checked and tested for COVID-19 regularly. Many families made the decision to isolate themselves from each other and the outside world as well.

Months passed, and the virus didn't slow. Every time people questioned whether or not the virus was real, coronavirus reminded us of its fury. Local governments had businesses on a yo-yo and opened and closed them with little explanation. The public struggled to figure out the logic behind the decisions as gyms and barbershops closed, while larger casinos, groceries, and department stores remained packed in large numbers. The same politics was played with schools, cities, churches, beaches, and more.

The one constant thing, despite it all, was how we still couldn't visit Mom. Her nursing home was only a few minutes from my home, however, no visits were permitted. Selfishly, I pondered ways to see her, but at this point, who was that benefitting? Mom was content, her home's draconian measures were working—zero cases. I couldn't be mad about that. We phoned, but that was mostly an exercise in futility: Mom was either sleeping or distant and disoriented.

As time went on, the home got a special phone for FaceTime, and we were finally able to see Mom. Aside from struggling with technology, Mom smiled more than she had in a long time.

Mom's medicines were routinely increased and changed

to keep her comfortable and prevent her from getting agitated. I know, because I received the calls. The nurses told me one night at her bedtime that Mom tried to kick all the residents and staff out of the building because the restaurant was closing.

I hoped she was thinking back to those nights we spent together at my restaurant. Sometimes she'd visit me near closing time, after finishing up with one of the elderly women she cared for. Always valuing cleanliness, she'd help me finish the nightly dishes or take the lead in mopping the floor. I'll never be able to repay her, but I'll always try. Back then, I tried to reciprocate by making potato skins or creating a unique vegetarian dish. Portabella mushroom caps were her favorite, and together we'd decide on spaghetti and meatballs, a fish sandwich, or hot sausage for Dad.

I was always glad to see Mom smile, but it filled me with emotions: happiness, anger, sadness, and so much guilt. I was a mess. Her sentences were garbled, and word usage was never quite right.

If I stood in front of a cloud, she would say, "What's that big green thing behind you?"

If I had on a red shirt, she would say, "That thing there is nice."

This was Mom, my hero, and I'm thankful every heartbreaking second for her. Guilt fills everyone who has a loved one with Alzheimer's, and my family is no different. We all had regrets, things we wish we had said or things we wish we hadn't. *Could we have done more,* and *are we doing enough.* The guilt is something loved ones keep within because we know we're lucky. My spouse lost her dad as a young woman, and I know so many who have lost loved ones prematurely. Wouldn't it be selfish for me to grieve a loss that hasn't happened yet? Aren't those facing this battle fortunate to still have our loved ones? There they are; we can see them, speak to them, and hold them. Yet, it feels like I lose my mom over and over. She's there, but she doesn't remember these stories, my children, or me. I grieve, but I do it in the shadows, and my heart breaks.

CHAPTER 19

LOOKING
FOR ANSWERS

EARLY SUMMER 2020

Mom saved a lot of papers, mail, and memories. That meant that when she moved into the home, we had to get her affairs in order. My sister, Dad, and I have spent many hours combing through Mom's memories looking for answers. We knew she had saved a few dollars, and the more we looked the more information we found. Random accounts with a few hundred dollars and retirement accounts with money she had saved for years working at our local thrift store turned up. It was our job to make sure that Mom was able to access and use every penny to make her comfortable. And we tried, but the whole process was beginning to feel like a sad and twisted treasure hunt.

Each step of the process was intense. In my mom's office she had two desks. She also had eight three-drawer filing cabinets, a closet, shelves, boxes on the floor, and a safe that Dad had to bust open with a hammer. In my sister's room were three more closets, a dresser, boxes under the bed, stacks on the floor, and all types of things she had hidden as her mind slipped. In my old room were boxes, two full closets, and another dresser. All of it was stuffed full.

This was the process, and so was a trip down memory lane. Mom kept everything she had deemed important since moving to Pennsylvania: our report cards, progress reports, resumés, and personal accomplishments. Mom didn't miss a thing. Indistinguishable Crayola drawings of mine, my sister's, and my children, all labeled with dates and ages. I'm grateful to have a mother who cared so much that she saved those memories for us.

I was also troubled, and the line between junk and gem often blurred. Old phone bills, business cards, magazines, and documents that should have been shredded long ago; in these things lay many of the answers we needed to help Mom. Little by little we battled the beast. Often the documents we found led to dead ends. Other times, we found accounts we didn't have access to. It took nearly a year to start getting answers, and there was always a roadblock.

Companies never tried to help; they just made us get more papers signed.

Mom worked her ass off for any savings she had, and when she needed it, we hit a brick wall. She worked nights and weekends and picked up odd jobs, but when she needed help, the financial institutions turned their backs. I called and called, and day after day I was cast aside. I called and emailed her ex-employer, but I guess Mom's years of service didn't warrant her a call.

After submitting all the necessary documents, the financial institutions still pushed back.

"Another week or two," they said. Or "We're waiting on the plan sponsor to review."

Always an excuse and never concerned. My mother had saved for a rainy day. Now it was pouring and no one cared. Week after week, the same bullshit responses. Never moved up the ladder, never made a priority.

Finally, after a wishy-washy conversation with a man who had little concern, I couldn't take it any longer.

They then asked, "Is there anything else?"

I responded, "Yes! I know you're recording this call, so I hope you will share it with your management team. My mom has dementia, and she needs this money for her care. I am befuddled by your company's lack of compassion or concern. My mom worked nights and weekends for over fifteen years, and when she needs it, your entire company turns its back. When some slick-talking sales-man convinced my mom to trust her retirement funds with your company, did they tell her if she got sick, tough

luck?" It wasn't the man on the phone's fault; however, he
didn't help either. That's just how it was.

CHAPTER 20

BRUTAL BUT BETTER

THE DOG DAYS OF SUMMER 2020

It's brutal not seeing my mom, but she's in a better place. My guilt is rising, but I try to convince myself Mom is safer in a home. She is healthier now and better off than the dark days before she fell and broke her hip. Mom's life had been full of bright colors, unique plants, and rooms bursting with sunlight. But not then. Those months were the toughest of this journey because Mom was disoriented most of the time. Covid-19 is terrible, but a year ago we were lost in the abyss. She sleeps a lot now, but back then she slept days on end. Even with help coming to assist, Mom was barely getting by. I tread lightly (out of respect), but hair, makeup, and hygiene were no longer under her control. When assistance was offered, or we tried to step in, she was aware enough to be offended.

Our mother would never have accepted a disheveled appearance, but that was what it had come to. We all tried to help: so many ways and so many times.

Dementia destroyed so many things my mom once loved. She prided herself on cleanliness yet filled her home with junk. She held on to things that were not worthy of her memory: Wendy's wrappers, old mail, and questionable laundry. My dad would spend all day putting out fires at work, and when he got home and made a pizza, often the pan and pizza were gone before he had a chance to eat it. Phones, pictures, presents, and mail were all hidden, forgotten about, or misplaced.

Looking through boxes at Mom's, I find old Christmas presents to Alissa and to Dom. One said, "To Mom, From Alissa." No matter how I tried to explain it, she didn't feel the gift was for her. I thought I should open it, and when I handed the gift to my mom, boy, was she angry.

One step forward and two steps back. You do one thing to try and help; instead, it causes problems elsewhere. A terrible domino effect. Everything my family did for her was out of love, but it's all left for interpretation. We all judge and tell ourselves we'd never let this or that happen to a loved one: *If I was in that position, I'd come to the rescue and save the day*.

After my search, I was flooded with memories, so I tried to make another FaceTime call to Mom. Each time, I was hopeful, but she looked at the phone and asked, "Who's that?"

Whoever handed her the phone had walked away. It was me and Mom, and a scowl. I smiled, showered her with kind words, and showed her some things around the house. She didn't say much, except for "Who's that?"

We lose Mom over and over again, and it hurts every time.

CHAPTER 21

INCHES SEEM LIKE MILES

LATE SUMMER 2020

Window visits, a cruel by-product of COVID-19. Since the elderly are at a higher risk, most were isolated from the outside world for their own protection. At Mom's home, a loved one could visit, but only if they stayed at least six feet away, wore a mask, and stood behind a glass divider. When Mom's memory-care home finally allowed this, I was torn over the right thing to do. I wanted to visit with my mom, hold her, hug her, let her know we cared, but Mom was comfortable, safe, and virus free. Were my own wants worth more than her safety?

My worry, as always, was that visiting may do more harm than good. When Mom was first admitted, we worried she wouldn't want to stay—and sometimes she tried to follow us out the door. Those visits were tough on my dad. Most of the time she slept or just kept watching television. When she did follow us, it wasn't because she missed home or knew who we were; it was just out of confusion.

Maybe this would be the day when you'd get a good twenty seconds. I knew she wouldn't know me, but you always carry the seed of hope.

During a FaceTime call, as we said our goodbyes, Mom looked directly into the phone's camera and said, "I miss you." Did she know me? Did she know I was her son? Did she know the person she was looking at loved her? These questions flooded my mind.

Some days, I called to talk to my mom and other days I called just to see if the staff had any updates on when we could visit her in person again. To my surprise, on this day's call, they told me they're allowing window visits.

"When can I come?" I asked.

"Anytime. Just call first so we can get her ready," they replied.

"Ten minutes?" I asked.

"We'll have her ready." She said other stuff, too, but my mind was already racing.

I hung up the phone and yelled up the stairs, "Maddie, do you want to go see Nanny?"

"When?"

"Two minutes. Brush your teeth!" I yelled.

To my surprise, she was ready quickly, wearing rubber boots, shorts, and a hoodie—an odd combo for summer, but I was glad to have the company. We jumped in my Jeep and were there in six minutes. It was up a hill, over a pair of uneven railroad tracks, past the Sheetz convenience store, a local barbershop, and the car wash on the right. Left at the light and up another hill. I always timed it. Always six minutes.

Finally. Our first window visit and, for the first time, face-to-face with my mother in months. I was nervous but comforted having my daughter by my side. In hindsight, I believe the emotional magnitude and unpredictability of a window visit with a loved one is too much for an eleven-year-old to process. This is the guilt I cling to. It wasn't fair for me to put her in the same hopeful position. Mom's memory had taken me from her long ago, and I knew she wouldn't know me. Still, I hung on to hope, and now my daughter hoped too.

Once parked at the home, Maddie and I grabbed our masks and hopped out of the Jeep. As we had done many times before, we crossed the blacktop parking lot and headed toward the elegantly painted double doors. There were twice as many signs as when I was last there: warnings reminding us of COVID-19 protocols and procedures to follow on the doors.

One of the administrators saw us wandering about as

she pushed in her code to enter and asked if we were there for a window visit. We said yes and told her who we were there to see. She directed us to a small bench near a fountain. The bench only sat one, and it was placed perpendicular to the window. In proper social distancing guidance, it was more than six feet away from the building.

Again, more signs, and they directed us to sit on the bench and wear our masks at all times. We had not seen Mom in months, and now only with masks, a sideways bench, through a window, and six feet away. Our anticipation grew, and we waited for the moment Mom would appear. I snapped a few pictures of Maddie sitting on the bench waiting for Nanny and hoped I would catch one of Mom when the window opened.

The window did open, about three inches. It was my friend Heather from high school who worked there and looked out for Mom. We chatted for a minute, and she said my mom would be over soon.

We waited, wondering if Mom was coming, nerves growing. Then behind the paneled window and dark screen, my mom appeared. Behind Mom was background noise. Behind us were speeding cars, large trucks, and other annoying road noise. The window was slightly cracked, and Mom moved her head toward the opening but was stopped when she tried to open it more.

We couldn't see her well through the small opening or the thick black screen, and Mom couldn't possibly have heard us through the muffle of our masks.

After about forty-five seconds of mostly unclear, uncomfortable, and inaudible conversation, Mom said something about finishing something before dinner. We nodded and smiled under our masks, hoping our eyes would convey our happiness, craving more engagement. But Mom turned her back and walked away.

Maddie and I stood by the window speechless, befuddled, waiting for Mom's return. We waited for her return longer than our visit and longer than it took us to drive there from our house. Mom never came back.

Maddie asked if Nan was coming back, and I tried my best to put some kind of positive fatherly spin on it. Whatever I said was bullshit.

We retreated to my Jeep, looking back to see if Mom had returned to the small opening, but it remained empty.

CHAPTER 22

I CAN'T LET GO

SEPTEMBER 2020

I found my Starting Lineup action figures while looking through my sister's old room where Mom had slept the last few years. I knew my mom hadn't thrown them out. I found many things: papers and pictures, food and candy, and hidden clothing that need not be discussed.

If I asked about them, she said, "I never saw them," or "Someone threw them out."

She was always defensive in matters of memory, but then sometimes an hour later she'd walk down the stairs with whatever thing we had asked about.

"Where'd Mom go?" we'd ask.

She wandered a lot, and we worried that someday she'd try and leave. One day, she told me a story about eating lunch with the ladies at the church. From the way she told the story, it seemed like she had just visited the church next door. She didn't go out, or did she?

Before I could drive, my mother loved to be out and

about. She drove me everywhere, without ever a complaint. If I wanted to go to a friend's, a skatepark, or the YMCA, she'd have me there. After getting cut from the seventh grade team and until I received my license at sixteen, Mom shuttled me to 6:00 a.m. men's basketball, noon games, and open gym at night.

When I was a sophomore in high school and somehow managed an invitation to an upperclassman's party, Mom had my back when I screwed it all up. This was the type of school party you see in the movies: teenagers acting rowdy, music blaring, cars parked on the lawn and up and down the street.

Early that evening I handwashed my car and polished my chrome rims. At about six o'clock I picked up my buddies, and we made our usual weekend stops: the mall, McDonald's, Speedy Mart, and a few lame attempts to buy beer. Once we decided it was a cool enough time to arrive, we hopped in my car and pumped up the bass. When we pulled on the block, it was like a teenage Disney World, and we had passes to the front of the line. We rolled in like rockstars, bass booming, and parked out front. We let the bass drop a few more times and then hopped out, feeling cool. Eyes turned our direction as the punch of the bass took the partygoers by surprise. For a moment, my friends and I were cool, and I was the man. We shut our doors and started off toward the house with the vibrations of bass accompanying us along the way.

After a few head bobs, I realized my keys were locked inside my running car. My options were slim: break the window, call a locksmith, or wait for a neighbor to call the cops and get the whole party busted. I chose "Option Mom." I called Mom from inside the house, and without hesitation she said, "I'm on the way."

I had never been to this kid's house—nor had Mom—and it was before GPS devices and cellphones, but she still made it in no time. Mom arrived and handed me the spare set of keys. She passed no judgment and offered no lecture—just a look.

I curved my partying and let my friends do their thing. I was cool for a night, thanks to Mom. And nobody was the wiser. Before her memory loss, regardless of the situation, Mom always offered me stability and wisdom.

Now we're in COVID-19 times, and my children have been stuck at home with Mom and Dad for nearly a year. Nan would be so proud of them; they're maturing and changing rapidly. She'd be sad that there were no games, concerts, or grandparent breakfasts at school. Most schools are teaching remotely, and my children haven't been in a school classroom for five straight days in nearly a year.

What would Mom have done? For one, she wouldn't let me hang my head. She'd offer encouragement, and I shall do the same. My role as a parent is more important than ever. I'm their example twenty-four hours a day, and I must be a good one. Even though I can't visit Mom, her lessons still guide me. Hopefully, I'm a strong role model and can allow my children to experience life with the same love, zest, and level of patience Mom bestowed upon me.

When this quarantine ends, I'm taking Mom to Chick-fil-A like we did before our world changed.

And, I'm saying thanks.

CHAPTER 23

MORE LOSS

2020 GRINDS ON

Mom deserved better than the hand she'd been dealt. Time and time again her dignity was stripped away— everything she loved, close enough to touch but still out of her reach. The proud beautician no longer cared about her hair. The woman we had known with closets and drawers packed with colorful and stylish clothes now let caregivers pick her outfits.

My children whom she spoiled with the "Nanny Train," she no longer knew.

On FaceTime calls, I'd talk about my daughter, Madilyn, by name. I'd have Madilyn stand beside me, and we'd talk to Nanny together.

"Mom, this is my daughter, Madilyn, and she's in sixth grade. Do you like her hair?" I'd ask.

When she replied quickly, our spirits were raised, but a second later she'd ask, "Who's that girl with you?"

Mom had so many pictures of us throughout her house

of when I was a teenager, I felt like I was famous.

Anyone who visited my parents' house had a full view of our childhood. Mom documented it all with pictures: pictures of me as a chubby boy in cowboy boots and a big hat, and pictures of my sister and me when we were in our awkward years wearing Jams, Skidz, pegged pants, or tie-dye, along with many unique hairstyles. I had Beatle cuts, spikes, buzzes, skater hair, and lines and images shaved. My sister was blessed with dyes and wonderfully tight perms forever cemented in photographs on my mother's wall.

When my children were born, Mom did the same. She found a home for every school picture and team photo: baseball, soccer, basketball, football, and Madilyn in a play as "Little Roo." My children loved seeing pictures of me with bowl haircuts and chubby cheeks, and I appreciated how proudly Mom displayed us all.

At the home, her room was filled with pictures and photo albums. Outside each resident's door was a special glass case full of their special mementos. This was to help guide residents back if they ever got lost. Mom's was full of her treasures, but without guidance, she typically ended up lying in another's bed.

Mom always treasured her photos; now she walked right by them.

I cherish more and more all the things she saved. This week my children and I visited Dad, and he offered us some trail mix covered in white chocolate to take home. Looking in his pantry for a baggie, I found a blue plastic lunchbox from 1984: Hulk Hogan, Rowdy Piper, and Ricky "The Dragon" Steamboat. Their muscles are bulging, and the picture is legendary, but inside is what gets to me: Mom's handwriting, *Dominick Domasky, Room #204*.

People always want vintage stuff, so I listed it on eBay. One guy kept lowballing me and even sent a personal note. Maybe I should just take the money; it's an old, plastic box. Yesterday, my son said he wanted it. Because of that, today I spent most of the morning figuring out how to delist an item. At lunch, I go upstairs to eat with my wife, a small dose of routine during a pandemic. Today, I was distant and ate my taco fast. On another day, the combination of Cool Ranch Doritos and leftover taco meat sprinkled with cheddar cheese and topped with salsa would have been magical, but today, not so much. I felt like I had to eat fast because I'm sick to my stomach thinking someone else will buy it before I get the job done. After lunch, I'm back to the computer, mission complete. We had a few bids, but this offer wins. A grandson likes wrestling and thinks it's cool that his grandmother kept it all those years. My children deserve some more good memories of Nan.

CHAPTER 24

2020 IS BREAKING ME

LOOKING BACK AT EARLY 2020

"My name is Sharon," my mom said, a stern crease between her brows.

She was talking to me. Startled, I collected my thoughts. What had I said that made her so angry? Casually, I had called her Mom; to her it was an insult. Increasingly, she was a child when we spoke. These thoughts seemed to last the longest when she spoke about her childhood. Her parents would have just asked her to do something; Dad was working, or he would be home soon. Her flashes of childhood memories tended to be the most precise.

One day I pulled up a Google Earth image from Las Cruses and showed it to Mom; she knew immediately it was her childhood home.

"Right there's where the swimming pool was." She pointed to the image. "The gate to the back was right over here. My brother dug a pool right there."

As Mom's memory went, I tried many things to help

her to remember. During the early stages, I could pick an ideal time of day—close to lunch and still light outside. As it progressed, those times were after lunch, still daylight, but in her favorite room. Mom had two rooms (sunrooms), and in each she grew beautiful plants. Mom had a green thumb and plants around the house, but here she was most comfortable. In those two rooms, more than any, Mom was closest to her former self. She'd sit with me and take part in conversation and rise to clip the leaves or remove the dead from a plant in need. If I asked about rooting plants or proper watering, she'd offer guidance on how I should care for mine. She would even make me cuttings from her favorite plants, which I was able to root in water through her teachings.

All my plants are precious, but the ones from Mom I adore. I bought us matching Venus flytraps, however, hers fell in the sink and died. Mine was mortally wounded when my children put french fries in its grasp. Little by little, death claimed my Venus flytrap. It's silly, but I was crushed when I lost it. Plants were one of my last connections with Mom, and I was losing those too.

Raising my voice and moving into Mom's personal space was a technique I often used to grab her attention. For years it worked. My tricks helped me gain precious time with my mom before she left again. These antics didn't make her happy, but I was always willing to accept a scowl or stern word for a moment with Mom.

The worst days were when she was unresponsive or when I couldn't get her to recall things that had excited her for years. Growing up in New Mexico, her favorite plants, the cats, those were my go-to's.

I asked, "When you were in Majorettes, what was the Rose Bowl Parade like?"

"I never did that."

When I saw Donald Trump on television I'd ask, "What do you think about him?"

She responded, "He's a nice guy."

I didn't want to stir her up; I just wanted another second with my mom, the mother who knew who I was. "Mom, what do you think about my haircut?" I asked.

"My name is Sharon!"

No Direction and No Help

More calls with Mom's financial companies. It's been months since I submitted all the papers they requested, and now they want more documents. My mom was such a dedicated employee during her years at the thrift store. Now when she needs them, I can't even get to someone live on the phone. My efforts are not helping; instead, I feel like a rudderless ship.

Can anyone hear me?

CHAPTER 25

THE PRESIDENT
HAS COVID

OCTOBER 2020

With thirty days until the election, the White House announced, "The president has COVID." Twenty-twenty was continuing its unpredictable ways. How could we keep Mom safe if the United States government and all the money and resources in the world couldn't keep our president safe?

Regardless of political affiliation, President Trump was a polarizing figure. People either believed he was the savior or the devil in disguise, and my mom was no exception. During 2020, he was in a hotly contested battle to maintain his position as commander in chief. Many people called it the battle for the soul of our nation. Long before President Trump's candidacy, Mom already disliked "The Donald." She wasn't political; she just didn't like Trump's brash persona.

Dad loved boxing, and the two had attended boxing matches across the country, including Las Vegas and Atlantic City, even staying in Trump's casinos more than once. Dad attended the legendary Tyson vs. Spinks bout, a ticket bought by Mom. The fight poster still hangs over the corner bar in their family room. Near the top, larger than the names of the fighters, the words Trump Casino loomed.

My dad read *Art of the Deal,* then lent it to me. It was one of the first books I read that was assigned by a teacher. Years later, President Trump was just part of pop culture. Appearances on Howard Stern and Oprah and buildings with the Trump name always present in our city skylines. Mom and Dad also watched the NBC show *Celebrity Apprentice* hosted by Donald Trump. I did too. On the show, people competed for an internship, and every week he sent one contestant packing—with his lips puckered, finger pointed, and the line, "You're fired!" Everyone I knew had a Trump impression.

Mom liked his ties. I know this because she complimented mine when I wore a suit. I often wore his brand-name ties because his ties made impressive knots; and at my favorite store, Burlington, they were always a deal. None of that mattered to Mom though. She didn't like his makeup, hair, or bravado.

Once he started becoming more political, my mom really let her thoughts fly. She was disappointed in his treatment of President Obama. Mom had worked for

Obama at the thrift store in Pittsburgh. Well, that's how *she* remembered it. People on television and in magazines were constantly appearing in her life. The meetings were full of details but completely false. Mom was getting more confused, but we didn't argue. As for Obama, she was there in his defense. Trump though, he made her mad. When she saw him on a magazine or on the television, her fuse lit. She'd say, "What's that 'Pumpkin Face' know? Look at that hair. Who does his creepy orange makeup?"

Trump got such a rise out of her, it was almost comical. Once she started, she went on and on; it was nearly impossible to change the subject. As with most children, from time to time we enjoy getting a rise out of our parents; I was guilty too. Mom's disdain for our future president provided many laughs.

As her Alzheimer's progressed, I was always searching for conversation topics. *What could I do or say that would hold her attention?* The plants and cats used to be my go-to, but now I just grasped for seconds.

Trump's on the television, so I'd ask her questions about the man on the screen. "Mom—" then I'd pause, hoping for a connection.

"Mom," I'd say, "what do you think about that guy?"

She said, "Him? He's a nice guy."

CHAPTER 26

THE TURNING LEAVES

LATE OCTOBER 2020

The holidays were coming, and it's been over seven months since we were allowed to see Mom face-to-face. I thought for sure the virus would be gone by summer, but now fall is here. The country is facing pandemic fatigue, but the virus is getting stronger. States that saw few cases early on are now having their emergency rooms overrun.

Near my mom's memory-care home there is a larger county-run retirement home. The Manor had little to no cases for months, and now staff and residents are under siege. Over a hundred have been infected, and the National Guard was called in. This place is less than half a mile from Mom, but Mom's place is still virus free.

I want to break the rules, but then I think to myself, "What if I have been exposed?"

I feel for the millions of seniors missing their families. Mom's comfortable, and we take solace. But what about the heartbroken, what are they to do? Their decision has been made for them: no visitors. And there goes what little connection I have.

There's news of a COVID-19 vaccine. They say it will be given to those at the highest risk. Pfizer is saying theirs is 90 percent effective. Another company says theirs is even better. The president says it will be distributed through Operation Warp Speed. We need a vaccine bad, each day a new high in the number of coronavirus cases in the United States—136,000, 138,000. Intensive care units are being overrun, and some hospital systems are being forced to cancel nonessential surgeries.

Another nursing home in my county had the National Guard called in. I worry every day that Mom's home will be overrun with this virus. It's surrounding us. My mind is spinning, and my guilt is off the charts. I question if we did what was right, or did we put Mom in a home and then abandon her. The facility is on lockdown, so she's safe—I guess. Physically safe. But what about emotionally? Are her needs being met the same way they would be if she was back home?

Other homes have allowed visitors in. I was jealous but conflicted. It now seems their residents are paying the highest price. I want Mom to be protected and safe, and her home still hasn't had one case. They're doing what they should be doing, putting their residents first. Mom even gained a few needed pounds—but how long can they keep the virus out?

Another FaceTime call, and Mom smiles. She's jovial. The conversation is all over the place, but she's *happy*. I walk about the house and show her the things behind me. My son's making scrambled eggs on the stove,, my daughter's in her purple bedroom, lying on her bed doing online schooling. My mom doesn't remember any of us but seems amused by the tour. It's something. She asks questions, and I continue looking for things to keep our conversation going. In the next room, my wife of nearly twenty years is sipping coffee. She's holding an oversized mug while working on the computer.

"Hello, Sharon. You look nice today," my wife says with a smile.

Something about her look, her voice, her smile, causes Mom to freeze. The silence was uncomfortable, but the energy was palpable. Liz and I both felt it, and we wondered afterward what my mom had been thinking at that moment. What did we stir up? Had she tried to grasp a fading memory?

On my television, the news channels show maps of the United States. The states filled in with red have rising COVID cases, and from coast to coast the map is red. Holiday gatherings are being altered, downsized, and outright canceled.

When Mom was healthy, she'd say, "Bull" (and spell "shit"). "I'm not going to live my life that way. Nobody's going to tell me where I can go." The sad thing is, Mom doesn't get to make those decisions anymore.

Mom would have hated COVID, the isolation, the division, the carnage.

I hate COVID-19; the vaccine can't come soon enough.

CHAPTER 27

DOES ANY OF IT MATTER?

NOVEMBER 3, 2020

It's election night, and Biden's out to an early lead. The polls had it as a potential landslide, but the state races are too close to call. Everything's different. COVID-19 concerns have more people mailing in ballots than ever before.

Nine, ten, eleven, and Biden's still leading, but incumbent President Donald Trump is coming on strong. Texas stayed red, and Florida supported Trump. Biden is projected to get the West, but neither has a clear path to two hundred seventy electoral votes.

At midnight, I tell my son he has to go to bed. We're still home in lockdown, but tomorrow is one of his scheduled days at school. He attends one day in person, and the next day through remote learning. My buddy Nick is here. He stopped by at eleven to watch the election. That's the type of thing you do in 2020.

Twelve, one, two, and the race is getting tighter. Neither candidate has a commanding lead. Biden speaks. It's late. He asks for patience and projects confidence. Pennsylvania, Michigan, Wisconsin, Trump's in the lead. Arizona, Nevada, Biden. But wait: Georgia is too close to call.

I'm invested, but does it matter? Here I am worrying about an election, but I am feeling guilty again. I should be focusing on my life, my family, and mom. When I was eighteen, I bought myself a used Chevy Blazer. I tinted the windows, bought new stereo equipment, rims, and made other cool modifications. When a buddy came back from college, he picked me up in his new Bravado; I sulked in jealousy.

When I told my dad about my buddy's nice car, he said, "How the hell does that affect you?"

Dad was a straight shooter, and maybe he was right. And maybe I shouldn't be so invested in a presidential race. The results will not turn lemons into lemonade. They won't change the events of 2020, nor will they cure Mom's dementia or give us back the months we were separated by COVID-19.

In the morning hours following election night, Trump declares victory with millions of votes left to be counted. The news networks remind us that the election has not been decided. The tension in the air is thick and unmistakable.

President Trump's margin is dwindling, and he calls on election officials to stop the count.

I sure wish I could talk to Mom about this election, the president's claims, and 2020.

When Mom caught me boasting or acting overconfident, she could not hide her displeasure. She would say, "Where's that pin? I'm going to pop your head like a balloon."

More votes were cast than in any other election in history, and the count continues for days. Trump accuses multiple states of fraud and puts the validity of the results in question.

"We won! We won big!" Trump exclaims, living up to his polarizing nature.

Joe Biden begins to pull ahead, and recounts confirm the results. Each day the margin of victory widens, and Joe Biden is elected the forty-sixth president. Many celebrate, dancing in the streets, and others feel robbed.

The country is divided once again. Maybe it's a good thing Mom wasn't here for this.

Can You Hold, Please?

———

I'm still battling with Mom's financial companies. The bills pile up, and I get put on hold again. Some days I wait an hour, and a recorded voice asks for my info. It says they will call me back, but they haven't yet. I doubt they ever will. When I get through to some companies, I'm so happy to hear a voice I nearly forget why I called. Each time, I tell the same story, and they request the same information.

What perturbed me the most is when they asked, "Is your mother there with you? Can she answer a few questions?"

"No, and she cannot. My mom isn't able to make these decisions," I reply.

They're confused and so am I. I've discussed Mom's situation for months with their representatives, but nothing changes. Each time I'm treated like a thief.

I have power of attorney and all the documentation they request. They still ask, "Can you put her on the phone?"

"My mom has dementia and is in a nursing home," I

reply sternly.

They dodge, duck, and weave. "Things are still processing. It will be five to seven business days."

My stress rises and another attempt to help my mother fails. Nothing changes. Our funds are dwindling, and her savings looks like it will remain untouched and hidden away.

CHAPTER 28

TURKEY DRIVE

THE WEEK BEFORE THANKSGIVING 2020

With the pandemic raging on, my friend Jim Aujay and I started a Turkey Drive to help families in need. My Dad saw we had taken on a big task and offered the deep freezer in his basement to me. I had underestimated the space needed to store six hundred pounds of turkeys, so I gladly accepted the space. Popsicles for my children, ice cream for Dad, and years of collecting everyone's favorites; that's what I found when preparing the space. Fried chicken, a large turkey, berries, nuts, and any snack you could think of.

It takes time and effort to maintain a fully stocked fridge, and Mom had three refrigerators and a deep freeze. I claimed the basement refrigerator as well and recruited my selfless wife to help me make room. Mom always had so much going on and did it so easily, but I was scrambling to get my head above water.

Each outdated item I pitched made me think of her. She prepared dinners, school lunches, kept a farmhouse clean, and helped my dad manage his business. She taxied me around town and picked up my friends too. All with a smile on her face.

Memories of my mother, I covet and cherish. Cleaning her deep freezer is cathartic. Every family favorite reminded me again and again of how much she loved my children, my sister, my dad, and me.

I find ingredients for the cheesecakes she so graciously made for my restaurant and special treats she stockpiled for the rest of our family.

All said, we're able to find space for over thirty turkeys. Feeling nostalgic, I ask Liz if we can tackle some closets. In Mom's bedroom, I find picture albums containing photos I've never seen. My parents' wedding album is in pristine condition. The pictures are in black and white, however, they jump off the page. Mom is beautiful, stunning, and so full of life. Dad's thinner than he's led me to believe and smiling from ear to ear. These photos unlock parts of my family history I knew nothing about, and I'm happy to uncover these memories. Mom wears glamorous dresses and her hair in a high beehive. Dad looks like a kid, smitten by his love for Mom.

Album after album, Mom and Dad are enjoying life. I see my grandfather and Dad shooting pool. My mom is on the edge of her seat looking on. I see Dad in his military uniform, and I see Mom proud of her man.

My wife is with me, and she's across the room diligently cleaning out a different closet. I'm not keeping up. I'm supposed to be cleaning and organizing, but each picture sends me deeper into my thoughts. There's still so much I don't know about my mother and father. Pictures I've never seen remind me of what I'm losing. Father Time marched forward, but I'm not ready to go just yet.

I pull photos out for Dad and others to keep. He says it's been years since he's seen them, and he gets lost in memory. "Here we were getting ready for a poker game; you had to dress up."

"Look at Mom here," I say.

Dad takes the photo and adjusts his glasses. Once again, he admires his wife.

I try to stay even keel, but I miss her so much. We all do. She's with us, but she isn't; and that's what breaks my heart.

CHAPTER 29

INSTITUTIONALIZED

EARLY DECEMBER 2020

The holidays are here, and the activity director from Mom's home reached out to me. I know the number by heart when I see it on my caller ID. She is creating memory books for each of the residents and wants to be sure they have something to open on Christmas. She let me know we could bring gifts, too, but because of COVID-19, they have to be dropped off five days early.

My sister sent some pictures, and I scoured around for some of my favorites: Mom bouncing on the trampoline in my backyard and smiling with my daughter, who was just a few years old at the time. I'm partial to the ones when I was young and chubby too—Mom always dressed me in cowboy boots and big ten-gallon hats. She and Dad all dressed up and ready for a night on the town was a good one too.

For a Christmas present, I chose two artificial plants for Mom, a red poinsettia and some succulents in a pretty pot. When Mom moved in, we tried to fill her room with some of her favorite plants, but we soon found houseplants can be dangerous to people with memory loss.

Mom's been away for almost a year, and the time hasn't healed anything. At home, her plants miss her dearly and most have lost their leaves. Dad tries his best, but the house is sterile now; it's missing her touch. The cats miss Mom too. Their farmhouse is no longer a sanctuary. We all miss her, and our guilt is apparent. We left Mom, and a pandemic hit. I stood on the sidelines as people debated the effectiveness of masks while witnessing Mom's nursing home be a perfect case study. They locked visitors out, their employees wore masks, and the residents stayed safe.

Twenty-twenty was a year full of complex challenges, and my family was no different than the millions who faced these same hardships. We all missed our loved ones, but during COVID the most effective way to protect them was distance. That meant hard choices and heartbreak.

My mother is past the point of knowing who's who, who I am, or how many days have passed since our last visit. She's comfortable and institutionalized. A doctor used that term with me soon after Mom's move, and I took offense. *Institutionalized* meant I'd take her out for the day, decorate her room just like home, and visit anytime I could—I'd never let it happen. I was knocked down routinely, and my efforts were nothing compared to the viciousness of Alzheimer's and the coronavirus.

Institutionalizing Mom kept her safe. Selfishly, I wanted to sneak in and visit her so many times. But the reality is, she was better off without me. I could call, FaceTime, or look through a dark screen at the window, but a simple hug was unattainable. I missed her touch.

The proverb is "Nana korobi, yaoki" and means "all down seven times, stand up eight."

We each faced hardship and tragedy in 2020, but please find hope knowing brighter days are ahead.

We had a snowstorm the last few days, and last night my wife pointed out all the snow covering the trees in our backyard. I commented about all the weight pine branches are able to hold. Then I told her how I climbed them as a kid. We climbed high and then walked out far on the limbs. We held on to the branch above, and when we did it right, it was like riding an escalator—we would lightly drop from high in the tree to ground level.

I had a dream last night about climbing these evergreen trees. I was with my lifelong friend, Anthony, at a Steelers game. The next thing I know, we were climbing these tall pines. I climbed high, walked out on a branch (as I had done as a boy) and gracefully rode it to the ground. I stepped off the branch into my parents' side yard. Standing there in her green coat and holding two bags was my mom. Her hair was black and beautifully styled—and I'm sure the bags she carried were full of gifts. I ran to her and hugged her tight. I awoke, and my heart was full of hope.

We'll see our loved ones again; and when we do, we'll hold on just a little longer and a lot tighter.

CHAPTER 30

HOPE

MID-DECEMBER 2020

The first Americans received COVID vaccinations, and millions of these vaccines are being shipped around the globe. The number of people vaccinated grows quickly, faster than the virus.

The president calls the speedy distribution of COVID vaccines Operation Warp Speed, and it couldn't come soon enough. Over a million lives have been lost around the world, and now over three hundred thousand in the United States. People still want to argue it's just the flu. If that's the case, then it's a flu that is ten times more deadly than what we see in a normal year. If it's all fake and media created, then why are so many hurting from lost loved ones?

I'm looking forward to a vaccine. In fact, I'd take all three. If possible, I may even bathe in it. I want to put this pandemic behind us. If me taking a shot helps keep my mom safe, then by all means, please sign me up.

America is a large and complex place, and we learn it

will take months to distribute all the shots. But there's hope. I know my mom and I will go out for lunch again. We'll hit the local Chick-fil-A, and I'll order her a chicken sandwich, a large lemonade, and make sure she has a few open ketchup packets for dipping her waffle fries. Together we'll walk the outdoor gardens of her care home, and over and over I'll attempt to retrieve more of her priceless memories—memories of my hero. Some she'll brokenly share, and others I'll uncover in dusty boxes.

Some dwell on the negative and cling to the pain, but I will focus on the good times and how much my mother loved me. I could write a thousand chapters, and it still wouldn't do justice to my mom's unconditional and undying love. She's an angel; and regardless of what the future holds, I will forever cherish her memory.

CHAPTER 31

HOPE CALLS

LATE DECEMBER 2020

I pick up the phone, and it's a woman from the thrift store in Atlanta.

She tells me, "Pittsburgh is out of my territory, but I got your voicemail, and I want to help."

I have been calling multiple companies on my mom's behalf, and each is a different fight. Whether it's the ambulance service or the financial institutions, they want Mom's money one way or another. They're more concerned with earning their points on my mom's meager investments than helping a woman in need.

Not today though. A compassionate woman from Georgia made a call to the Pittsburgh offices on my behalf. A woman I never met went above and beyond for a woman she never met. She gives me a number to dial and words of encouragement. I can't help but think that's what my mother would have done. They would have been fast friends, I'm sure.

———

And now there's hope.

I dial the phone while sitting in front of my computer. It's on speaker, so I continue to work away. I hear the same list of options I've heard over fifty times. I select option two. Account number, date of birth, confirm the last four digits of the social. The music plays. I'm on hold again. I want to scream: it's been eleven months of this.

A representative answers, "How can I help you?"

I go through the cycle again.

The representative says, "How can we help you, Mr. Domasky?"

I'm shocked they know my name. They're pleasant. The representative tells me I am listed as the power of attorney. There's no pushback or disconnected calls. She helps me, and I finally have access.

There's more work to do, but I'm seeing some progress. The weight on my shoulders lessens, and for today, Mom wins.

CHAPTER 32

COVID-19 IS GETTING CLOSER

JANUARY 1ST, 2021

I wish I could say Mom's wins mounted, but I'm notified there's a COVID-19 case at her nursing home. It's only one, but somehow the ugly virus has found its way in. Over four hundred thousand Americans have died now, and the virus seems to be getting stronger. Some argue it's just the flu and all made up, but each day more people become infected, and doubters turn into believers.

I went to my first COVID-19-related funeral this week. She was a healthy woman with many years of life ahead. She raised a great son, and they were very close. It's heartbreaking. Everyone I know seems to have a family member infected. If you go out without a mask, research is showing you are at higher risk, but distrust is everywhere. Another one of my friends lost her mom to the virus. She pleads to all who will listen to take this virus seriously and admits that she and her mother did not.

I'm doing some film work, and they test me three days

a week. On the weeks we film, it's five days a week. We wear masks, shields, stand six feet apart, sanitize repeatedly, and take regular temperature checks. Some days, it's only mildly uncomfortable; others, I pull away from the test administrator and wince in pain—I swear they've touched my brain. I've had over thirty tests now.

Poor Mom; she has to take weekly COVID tests now too. The tests are uncomfortable, and the residents don't understand why they're necessary. My mom bruises from the slightest touch; I can only hope they're being gentle. Ten months that staff kept the outside world out, but the virus is relentless. Retirement was supposed to be simple, the golden years: watching television, playing with the grandchildren, taking trips, and lots of naps. Instead, Mom is locked away with a mind at rest.

After a recent daydream, I was thinking about how my mom never got sick. Most winters, people get colds or the flu. Not Mom. Mom was bionic, our protector; and if sickness came, she prepared us warm chicken noodle soup with extra broth. For every ailment, Mom had a remedy. She always found a reason for me to gargle with warm salt water or drink Donald Duck brand orange juice.

She seldom rested. Maybe a little television—Dallas or Miami Vice—or a magazine here or there. But she was more active than any of us. Mom stayed up later and got up earlier. In my grandest attempts, my home will never be as tidy as one kept by Mom. Truth be told, if we didn't hang our shirts or fold the clothes in our drawers, Mom would be furious. She held us to the highest standards. Not because she was mean, but because she believed we were capable of so much.

Mom was a dreamer, and it seemed that in her dreams, she always put us first. Mom believed in our potential, and she believed in hope and possibility.

By witnessing Mom's grace and persistence, I'm confident we all have what it takes to overcome any challenge we are faced with.

CHAPTER 33

IT'S ALWAYS DARKEST BEFORE DAWN

WEEK 2 OF JANUARY 2021

After living in fear for months, I got the dreaded call—my mom tested positive for COVID-19. How shitty of a son am I? I pushed taking her out of her home, and now her life is in danger. A vaccine is here, but the roll-out is behind schedule. As if Mom hasn't been through enough, now she has this to deal with. She's hurting, and we're still not allowed to visit. I've been checking in daily. When they put her on camera, I hear her cough. It's deep, and it shakes her chest. Most days she sleeps more than usual. After two weeks, it is clear the virus has taken a toll on her.

Our country is hurting too. Yesterday, we witnessed the unrest and division caused by the ongoing crisis come to a climax. There was an attack on democracy by angry protestors. Our president called on his supporters to be strong and not weak. Under his directive—or confused by his words—an angry mob of Americans marched down the pristine streets of Washington D.C. and attacked the hallowed United States Capitol Building. A building once believed to be impenetrable was breached, and rioting ensued. Damage was done, people were hurt, and lives were lost. The building was locked down, and there was a delay in election proceedings.

Our country was shaken to its core; but resolute, congress reconvened late in the evening and worked until dawn. The electoral votes were counted, and Vice President Pence declared Joe Biden the undisputed winner of the presidential election. In the days that followed, the world learned of many heroes and cowards on this day.

I get a call from the therapist. She says, "Your mom is weak, but it looks like she's getting better."

Forever a fighter, Mom recovers. A few days later, my phone rings again. It's a nurse from the care home, and we schedule Mom for her first dose of the vaccine. It looks like the worst days of COVID-19 are behind her. The country is beginning to heal as well.

CHAPTER 34

HOPE IS WITH YOU

FEBRUARY 2021

"You can accomplish your wildest dreams." My mom ingrained that message in my DNA.

What a special gift to share with a loved one, the gift of hope and possibility. These are two beliefs that I have clung to during my mom's illness.

On FaceTime calls, her words are typically jumbled and thoughts scrambled, but every so often, as we ended a call, she'd say, "I miss you." Maybe it was habit, but for a few seconds here and there, my heart tells me she knew I was her son. These are the seeds of hope that I hang on to. Maybe Mom will have a good day or even a good moment. Maybe there will be a vaccine for memory loss, just like the ones being developed for COVID-19. If so, Mom and others like her could be healed, and memory loss would be a thing of the past.

My friend Matt Burnsworth is a four-time cancer survivor who talks openly about knocking on death's door. Matt shared a quote with me from a surgeon, Dr. Sugarbaker, whom he credits with saving his life.

"Hope plus anything equals possible."—Dr. Sugarbaker.

Over four hundred thousand Americans have lost their lives to COVID-19, but this quote fills a void in my heart, and I return to it often. The vaccine is en route, and I saw Mom through the window again. She was behind a closed window and dark screen, but I could still see her beauty. Her skin was clear and smoother than I remembered, and her smile was brighter than it had been in years. Mom looked good despite it all.

I tried to snap a picture; however, the dark screen and window didn't do her justice.

We tried to talk through a closed window, but she couldn't hear me, and I couldn't hear her. Nothing about Alzheimer's and COVID-19's impact was simple. After a few minutes, a caregiver held a phone to the window, and there was a label on the back with a phone number to call. I called, and they connected Mom and me through speakerphone. She talked about things she could see from the window, and I tried my best to make her smile. There was feedback on the line—the kind that happens when phones are too close—and the call was muffled. But it was a win. I saw Mom, and she was comfortable and safe.

After a few minutes, Mom abruptly walked away, and another resident moved forward and picked up the telephone. I looked at her and she studied me, and neither of us said a word. I was a stranger to both her and my mother. Like my mother, she was uninterested in my presence and also turned away. The woman located my mom and followed her back to the community room.

I stood outside alone.

CHAPTER 35

YIN AND YANG

MARCH 11TH, 2021

On the morning news, I see a large stimulus bill is passed. It's over six hundred pages, so I don't know how to respond. There's news about Prince Harry and wife Meghan and reports about the royal scandal. My daughter is getting ready to catch the bus and talks at a feverish pace. I pause the television as she updates my wife and me on all things TikTok. She heads outside to catch the bus, and I take a deep breath. I resume the show, and the newscasters discuss the details of the stimulus plan. Some say it's too big, and others say it's not enough. I fill myself with iced coffee and lose interest in the subject. As my mind wanders, I catch the words I've been waiting to hear since last March: the president says it's okay to visit people in nursing homes.

My head drops into my hands, and I'm overcome with joy. I try to collect myself, but I can't; the journey's been too long. My wife comes to my side to comfort me, but I'm not ready to lift my head. I need more time.

Moments later, I decide to run to the grocery store. As

I start my car, I see the nursing home's number on my Caller ID. The voice says, "Dominick, we are going to start allowing visitors on the 15th."

I miss Mom so badly, but instead, I volunteer my dad. He deserves it more than me. Tammy, the administrator, said we could both go. I ask about the process, and she says, "You're the first one I've called."

I try to answer but I can't. Again, I'm overcome with emotion. Finally, I get something sensible out, and Tammy shares the schedule. I brokenly asked for eleven o'clock. She puts me on the schedule, and I do my best to say thank you. Again, I can't compose myself, but neither can Tammy. We sit in silence but say more to each other than we ever have.

MARCH 12TH, 2021

My phone rings, and it's the nursing home again. It's Tammy, and she is soft-spoken, hesitant to speak and careful with her words. I already know it's bad news. She says, "A resident that recently checked into the hospital has tested positive for COVID-19." Based on government protocols, it is treated as a new case, and all visits are off."

I think Tammy expected me to lash out. But I didn't, and I couldn't; it's not their fault.

My hug would have to wait.

CHAPTER 36

THE WARMEST EMBRACE

MARCH 15TH, 2021

The day I was supposed to see Mom; however, the visit was canceled.

MARCH 19TH, 2021

I check my notifications, and I see a missed call from Mom's home. My stomach drops. When I call back, they let me know they'll be scheduling visits again next week. We'll have to wait another few days.

MARCH 20TH, 2021

The morning show I am watching reports that the pandemic has been going on for a year. They replay early clips from 2020 talking about COVID-19 coming to the

United States and the possibility of a lockdown. They show the explosion of cases and the effects it's had on our lives: businesses shuttered, social division, political division, mental health effects, students homeschooling, and too much death.

Minutes later, my wife and I begin our walk, and we see hundreds of cars parked in the nearby college's parking lot. This lot has been mostly empty for a year. Today, it is full of life; there is a vaccine clinic being held. Birds are chirping, and it's the first day of spring.

MARCH 22ND, 2021

It's 9:00 a.m., and I see those familiar digits: 5711. It's Tammy, and I schedule a visit for the next day: me and Dad with Mom.

MARCH 23RD, 2021

I wake up before my alarm clock. This is the day I've been thinking about for over a year. Our visit with Mom is scheduled for one thirty, and I'm nervous all day. In my mind, I try to lower expectations of what the visit will hold. All of us with loved ones ill or hurting hold on to hope. We're human.

Dad and I meet in the parking lot and walk in together. All the signs that have kept visitors out for over a year are gone. We're welcomed in by the staff, and their spirits are high. Dad and I are led to a conference room. We're the first visitors in a year. We sit around a large table and wait for them to bring my mother out.

Through the double door she comes, assisted by a caregiver. Her hair is grayer, but she looks healthy. She stops and sits on a bench, her limp still pretty bad. Mom is fifteen feet away with no screen or window between us. I can't believe it's been a year.

As they come closer, Mom sees me, and the staff asks if she knows who I am.

She responds, "My brother."

And I respond, "You're right."

Tammy asks if I'm the one she has been talking to on the phone.

"Yes," I said with a smile.

We all understood Mom needed unconditional love and not correction. Next, Dad asked about hugging his wife and whether or not we could take our masks down to let Mom see our faces.

Tammy shakes her head no.

As she exits the room, she looks back one last time toward my dad and me and softly says, "You must keep your masks up and remain six feet away, but I'll be out here for the next thirty minutes."

CLOSING

I didn't write this book to chronicle 2020, COVID-19, or a presidential election. My goal was to give a voice to Alzheimer's. I wanted you to meet and get to know my hero, Sharon K. Domasky. My objective was to share her story with the world, the memories stolen, the beautiful, the ugly, and the cruel truths only those who have faced this disease know. Mom's battle with memory loss collided head-on with 2020, and both have been tough. Alzheimer's is a disease that affects all parts of a family unit and all those involved. We each grieve and respond to these challenges differently, but we must understand that we are not alone.

I am thankful to those who comforted me. I am grateful to everyone who shared their journey of Alzheimer's and dementia with me. It is you who picked me up when I was at my lowest.

I learned adversity is a great teacher if we heed its lessons. Here are a few things I learned:

Don't keep your feelings bottled up; support is near.

Live this day like it is your last, as tomorrow is not promised.

Say thank you, and do it more.

Say "I love you" daily.

I'd say our lives can't change in a moment, but that's not true; they *do* change.

My mom's story is so much more than "victim of disease." She is a kindhearted and beautiful woman who fell in love with a young and handsome military policeman in Las Cruces, New Mexico. That woman moved across the country to Pennsylvania, started a family, traveled the world, and made everyone she encountered feel special. I was one of the lucky ones she lifted the most, receiving a lifetime of her love. I have spent years writing and publishing books, but in no way was I prepared to describe my mom's inner light or articulate what she means to me. Sharon K. Domasky is so much more than I am capable of expressing.

In these pages, it would have been disingenuous for me to share only the good times. Alzheimer's has been—and is—a world of shit. Mom's battle with Alzheimer's hasn't been cute like it's depicted on television and in movies. Mom was robbed of her dignity and left without a voice. Hopefully, this book can help give a voice to those battling memory loss and the families hurting who are doing their best to cope.

Remember friends, as long as you believe, love, and never give up—there is always hope.

You are not alone.

ABOUT THE AUTHOR

Dominick Domasky is an inspirational author, storyteller, and founder of the publishing platform Motivation Champs. Dominick is the author of the books *The Journey of a Grunt*, *How to Write a Book in 2020*, and creator and coauthor of the hit book *Go Ask Your Dad*. His greatest accomplishments are his two children; and he aspires to be the best father, friend, husband, and son he can be.

Dominick and Motivation Champs share inspiration, smiles, and positivity 24-7, and help others do the same. This mission is accomplished through publishing, screenwriting, a large social media footprint, in-person events, and work with nonprofits. Dominick and his son, cameraman Cameron, are the creators of a web series *Discovering Inspiration*, where they spotlight inspiring people and organizations.

Dominick can be contacted for events, speaking engagements, or publishing opportunities at www.motivationchamps.com He can be found daily @MotivationChamps.